THE ONE OF THE EMERALD TABLET

Friend Christina Root Dec 17 2016

So many fond memories of you and your family.

Remember me through these pages love!

THE ONE
of the Emerald Tablet

Illuminating Ancient Cryptic Truths

Anna Lups, MBChB, MD

SteinerBooks | 2017

2017
SteinerBooks
An imprint of Anthroposophic Press, Inc.
610 Main St., Great Barrington, MA 01230
www.steinerbooks.org

Cover painting: Liane Collot d'Herbois (1907–1999)
Book design: Anna Lups, Peter Pupator, and Jens Jensen
Author photo © by Dyana van Campen (dyanacamera.com)
Cover design: Jens Jensen

Library of Congress Control Number: 2016958702
ISBN: 978-1-62148-164-5 (paperback)
ISBN: 978-1-62148-165-2 (ebook)

Printed in the United States of America

Contents

Prologue . . . vii
Introduction . . . x
Gallery of the Child Artist . . . 1
Process of Consolidation . . . 9
DROP-formation . . . 10
Gesture of Dispersion . . . 16
Gesture of Consolidation . . . 17
The Initiation of Kings . . . 19
The Tabula Smaragdina . . . 21
Quality of Numbers . . . 23
One—the Sophia . . . 23
Twofold . . . 24
Threefold . . . 28
Fourfold . . . 29
Fivefold . . . 30
Sixfold: Contribution of Speech . . . 33
Sevenfold—Life on Earth . . . 34
Sound A . . . 35
Alchemy as the First Science . . . 39
Processes in Nature . . . 40
Threefold Function in the Human Form . . . 42
Three Kings . . . 43
Alchemical Equipment . . . 45
The Path of Initiation for the Alchemist . . . 46
Sound E . . . 47
History of the Gnostic Myth . . . 49
Soul Genesis . . . 51
Evolution of the Soul-Psyche . . . 52
Physical Incarnation—Soma . . . 53
Embryogenesis: Incarnation of The One . . . 54
The Birthing of the Child . . . 68
Sound I . . . 71
Seven-year Phases in Child Maturation . . . 76
Story of the Unbeliever . . . 78
Story of the Believer . . . 86
Sound O . . . 91
The Experience in O for a Person on Earth . . . 96
Gender . . . 97
Sex, Love, and the Future of Humanity . . . 99
Being a Woman . . . 101
Being a Mother . . . 105
The Act of Marriage . . . 108
As Lover . . . 110
The Credo . . . 110
Being a Doctor . . . 111
Sound U . . . 115
The Physical Organization, Myth, and the Vertical Plane . . . 117
Etheric Organization and Fairytales . . . 119
The Liver . . . 121
The Lung . . . 122
The Kidney . . . 124
The Heart . . . 126
The Astral Organization: The Parable . . . 127
The "I" Organization: The Legend . . . 130
Epilogue . . . 133
References and Recommended Reading . . . 135
Acknowledgments . . . 136
List of Plates . . . 137

Dedicated to Matthea and Max—the next generation

Prologue

This book has become mainly autobiographical, written from meetings with some of my patients over the fifty years I was in a position of confidence and guiding their health issues. Born in the Netherlands four years before World War II and living for five years under German occupation, my primary education was scanty and sporadic. Soon after the war, my family immigrated to South Africa, where I received secondary schooling and, subsequently, my degree as a physician. In 1959, at the early age of twenty-three, "the responsibility for" was bestowed on those taking home a MBChB degree. This was an English double Bachelor's Degree in medicine and surgery, allowing the "holder" to practice medicine in all English protectorates throughout the world.

Politics in South Africa was turbulent. Apartheid increased the schism between skin colors, as well as between the haves and have-nots. Because there was no future for me in that environment, I considered emigrating to the U.S. I received papers to do so in 1963. While awaiting citizenship status, I gathered practical experience in the rural areas of The Transkei, South Africa. As a Dutch citizen back in the Netherlands, I had undertaken a two-and-a-half-year training in cardiology at the university where my parents had received their medical degrees. In mid-1963, I received the official documents as a U.S. immigrant. No threats of expulsion, no green card; America here I come!

The popular musical opera by Leonard Bernstein, *West Side Story,* reverberated in my heart. In contrast to South Africa, the United States is the country that receives all with open arms. Being a foreigner was special, and the somewhat European accent added cachet when meeting new people. From the moment of setting foot on American soil, I felt American! This country possesses an underlying hospitality that validates the work of an industrious person.

I accumulated many experiences during the following four years: residency in internal medicine; moonlighting in a busy inner-city emergency room; a serious relationship with a partner; and pregnancy and motherhood. It all precipitated in a decision to strive toward independence.

My search for a home in a quiet, bucolic environment was completed when I became the owner of a ranch-style house nestled in the quiet hamlet of Hillsdale, Columbia County, New York. As a single mother, I was now on my own. The idea of "hanging my shingle" made me ebullient; nothing could deter me in my search for an individual expression and following a dream. As an immigrant, family ties were absent, but connecting with the wholesome witty local citizens was a boon to my life and a constant source of inspiration for stories I would accumulate. My son made friends and was not shy about crawling over the snow three houses down the street to pursue his own independence. Skiing in the winter was our favorite pastime; injuries, fractures, and such could not keep us away from the slopes, which were just around the corner from our home.

During the next ten years my practice became established, and privileges in the local hospital enabled me to extend influence on a broader scale of medical disciplines, which included psychiatry, prenatal care, and birthing. I felt a deep connection with the mothers in their intuitive desire for something altogether different in their experience of motherhood. It was "hippy" culture, but they were certainly successful in inaugurating the new movement of natural childbirth, home deliveries, water births, breast-feeding, and rejection of circumcision. These were all impulses I was willing to encourage, and I was able to assist with at least a hundred births in the ten years that followed. Even now, twenty odd years after that period, I meet young people in the area who know that I was present at their births in a very intimate way. The continuum of medical concern gives them the trust that healthcare can be human.

Mental health care in Columbia County during the 1970s was an extraordinarily inadequate system. The old guard of physicians must have believed that little could be done for a family member who was derailed, and confining them to the mental hospital in Wassaic, New York, was not popular. A diagnosis of mental Illness could stigmatize, and therefor was not often made. It was even suggested that mental disease did not exist in Columbia County. The existence of a mental health society for lay people allowed me to facilitate greater awareness among the local population. Popular songs such as Don McLean's ode to Vincent van Gogh, who cut off his ear a year before his suicide, stirred the hearts of fathers and mothers who needed to know that a greater group of people in similar circumstances did support one another in times of need. My three-year service on the board of that society saw a change in the habit of placing responsibility on the family, as alcoholism and depression were increasingly identified as health problems, and adequate protection was legislated for suffering family members. Changes were in the air.

The acquisition of a second home just opposite the emergency entrance of the hospital in Hudson, New York, enabled a greater dedication to the population of the county. I had a strong conviction that the city of Hudson was an architectural treasure in spite of the exodus of most business on the main street. Liberty Medical Arts, as I named my practice located on Columbia Street, was then able to sponsor lectures on local medicinal plants, homeopathy, and holistic medicine. One of the largest events was an exhibit of local painters and their magnificent works. The old flour mill still stood just behind the St. Charles Hotel. It was an impressive building with gorgeous spaces for hangings and other art. The artist Fred Harris in particular worked on the space for many days to create a truly artistic event.

At the age of forty-two, a subtle change in my thought and deeds became evident. I heard lectures by Otto Wolff, MD, that shook me to the core. His expertise was gleaned from a spiritual path called Anthroposophy, begun by Rudolf Steiner in the early 1900s. It is an esoteric Christian offshoot from Theosophy. Indeed Dr. Steiner, who had obtained a doctorate in philosophy ten years earlier, was asked in 1902 to lead the Theosophical branch in Germany as its president. An expert on Goethe's writings—both literary and scientific—gave Dr. Steiner the authority to form opinions on modern science and literature. I was introduced to a completely different world of thought, recognizing familiar memories and mental pictures for which I lacked a language. It was exciting and grounded me with a stubbornness to stand by my authenticity. Answers to questions flooded my consciousness. Questions about myself arose: Who am I? Where are my beginning and my end? Is the Earth the only planet with life? Do we live only once? What is the distinction between a person and an individual? Are we alone? And, given my Dutch Reformed indoctrination, who is the Christ?

We are all pigeonholed in the Western society. Stepping out of such constraints takes courage, desire, curiosity, and confidence. Having an abundance of energy, I could call that period a conversion of sorts. I was willing to convert my practice to a discipline in keeping with my spiritual path. As a physician, one could still introduce a spiritual aspect, understanding that my patients needed to sense my interest in their overall goals in life and their dignity of social position, while also recognizing where they had gotten stuck in their individual biographies (a source for their illnesses), and being able to guide them to the possibility of self-healing.

The following years were instrumental in completing the dream I had imagined since childhood. The times that my parents exposed me to farm life were the happiest. Gathering eggs, milking with the farmer, bottle-feeding the calves, and cleaning and raking—I never had enough. Did I still carry fear for the unrest and deprivation of war itself? Deep down, I knew that being true to spiritual lawfulness meant giving up self-directed desires, obedience to the greater good, and familiarity with poverty. Didn't my farmer family live much more simply, and weren't they profoundly happy?

I purchased an orchard just south of Olana, the estate of the nineteenth-century artist Frederic Church, after divesting the ranch in Hillsdale. This was the first step toward creating a space where physical and mental disciplines could be harnessed to strengthen the will. I christened it *Pleroma,* a Greek word meaning "paradise," or "fullness of the Divine." Furthermore, such a lifestyle shared with patients could create a healing environment in which both the soil (through the practice of biodynamic agricultural methods) and the human soul would be given a chance to become balanced. I was inspired by the work of an anonymous writer, *Meditations on the Tarot*. A study of this text made it clear that innate wisdom is not acquired but already exists deep within all of us. How can we make ourselves listen?

Then and now—thirty years into this biography I started the farm at the age of fifty, and only now can I consider letting go of it as it is. Many patients have experienced the magic of nature bestowing a bounty of gifts and insights on them. What happens here on the farm lives on; it is authentic and inspiring, and it creates in all of us love for life, freedom, and hope that life lived is not in vain. Indelible impressions have accumulated throughout fifty years of exercising the gift of sharing and learning from both young and old. Those who bore the burden of altering my life have filled me with unforgettable stories.

Most astounding for me as a physician has been to experience the revolution in healthcare—issues of control over life and death, the subtle change toward financial gain so many persons in our field support, and the explosive development in the field of pharmacological chemistry. In general, modern healthcare lacks a spiritual context for patients as individuals, yet patients are searching for meaning in their infirmities in a time when beliefs in the temporal and infinite existences collide. For a physician who can follow an individual spiritual practice, opportunities to meet the patient as an individual in contrast to just another person becomes a prerogative that can never be taken lightly. These become the highlights in a medical career and opportunities to share concepts of infinity and the laws of reincarnation with those people. Hope is connected to the future. These stories are interwoven and presented throughout the book.

Anna Lups, September 2016

Introduction

Spiritual Science, as begun in the early twentieth century by Rudolf Steiner, has planted many seeds in our lives. This text endeavors to shed knowledge on the fact of spirit-human incarnation and immortality. Many disciplines, occult and open, ancient and modern, are referenced herein. A base understanding of Anthroposophy, alchemy, biology, and the arts will allow the reader faster understanding of the concepts presented.

Inspiration from the work of the "Child Artist" is the genesis of this text. For many hours I have tasked myself with the intuition to form many imaginations of his work. Accordingly this text starts with a presentation of the Child Artist's work unadulterated. As fragments from these drawings are presented I will reference the reader back to the original plate, now with a unfolding imagination in context with the specific concept presented.

This book is dedicated also to that Child Artist. After two visits he decided of his own free will not to return. My dedication comes from gratefulness to the younger generation—those who carry knowledge of so much and are unable to make it understood.

Medical science medicates effectively but without real understanding of what happens to the life process of a patient. Authenticity in the young is difficult to accept but the most precious aspect in our society.

Considerable insight into the *Tabula Smaragdina* (Emerald Tablet) was derived during the writing of this book. Indeed I discovered that the Child Artist spoke the Alchemical language. This dovetailed well with my own reading and investigations in life. This most sacred of texts shaped the outcome and model for **The One**. I attribute the Emerald Tablet to Hermes Trismegistus, the half-god, half-human of lore (Thoth). Originally translated from the Latin version, I have included it in this writing.

Evolution plays a dynamic, formative force in nature. The folding of sheaths, like a blanket, over and over again, is a theme that is discussed in detail. Onefold, twofold, threefold—this will go on forever. In this text I stop at the sevenfold, the place at which the life process plays a formative role in human evolution.

Understanding the Sophia and the Christ as highly developed spiritual beings who will supersede the experiences of the five senses on Earth will be a future task. The evolution of the human being is interwoven with these God-beings, and "doing it alone" is not their itinerary. More often They will announce themselves, make requests resulting in mental and even cellular changes for our growth and development.

Certainly this book is about **The One**. My use of bold is intentional and compulsive throughout the text. This intentionality should evoke the reader's personal concept of self, transcendent from time. Simply stated, **The One** is the timeless Spirit-being, the identity that can incarnate on Earth multiple times. **The One** is not to be confused with the "I" of the soul life. The use of "I" is also intentional and consistent. The "I" is the soul's response to stimulation and memories accumulated—the Jungian and Freudian Ego. The term *old soul* comes to mind as a case in which multiple incarnations have allowed **The One** to shine into the soul life as a palpable presence.

Likewise the use of *Gaya* (*Gaia*) and *Sophia* requires definition. Gaya is the mythical goddess associated with the Earth. Sophia (wisdom) can be best described in this text as the soul experience of Gaya. In a Gnostic sense Sophia is more palpable and accessible to human beings on Earth.

A discussion of the nomenclature and pronunciation of the vowel sounds is merited. The European and English languages differ, as do colloquial pronunciation and dialects. The same letter having different sounds in context with consonants is also of interest. For example the word amen can have both an "ah" or an "ey," depending on contextual usage. It is interesting to feel how the same word pronounced differently can affect the human differently. Language is a formative process. In this text, I use only English pronunciation. To avoid confusion, the following letters are used for the corresponding vowel sounds. The reader is encouraged to sound out each of the vowels in times of reflection, as well as when encountering them in the text.

Letter	**Pronunciation**	**Examples**
A	ah	amen, hallelujah
E	ey	craze, change
I	ee, ii	team, repeat
O	oo	close, hope,
U	uu	universe, community

I encourage the reader to keep a separate notebook to record impressions during the reading of the text. It is always important to write and speak important truths. Once written these impressions, questions, or new thoughts must be pondered, and at last spoken in a hushed breath. Truths when spoken shape and mold the soul in health. Regardless of your religious or educational background, your profession or hobbies, it is my hope that this book will encourage you to think, feel, and will out of your **One**.

Finally this book when read and understood is a process of initiation—in the becoming. It encourages the reader to become aware—"you are more than who you think you are." The most important thing to bring is your sense of humor, light, and curiosity, for that is the stimulus of imagination

"When I was fifteen I discovered something inside myself.

I discovered that what was inside of me was infinite
That one can go down to the bottom of one's soul
And keep reaching and reaching and reaching.

Not only me, but everybody was like that!

The discovery of a quality of super-human power
Unfathomable majesty, infinite existence was part of me, my "I AM,"
With this knowing I could enter my life, my dance"

Scripted from a play *Without a Word*
words spoken by the lead ballerina Chrissie in the movie *One Last Dance*

Gallery of the Child Artist

During my role as school physician in the late nineties (*September 1998*) I was introduced to a kindergartener with extraordinary drawing capacities. I will refer to him hence as the Child Artist, out of respect for his talent to guide us in discoveries that far surpass the natural scientific module. His drawings, detailed, orderly, of exceptional accuracy, beauty, and purity, convinced me as an observer, that here was a story needing to be explored. It was a gift for me to explore the mystery behind these drawings, though they were not penetrated with an adult consciousness.

The Child Artist and I were exchanging a weekly dialogue with each other only for a period of three months. During the short period I could work with him, he gave me no indication as to the meaning of the beautiful representations he shared with me. There were no stories connected with any drawings. I witnessed him draw, using colors as he saw fit. There were at no time any questioning or other interferences from an adult out of fear that this could influence the pure inspirational artistic flow. The drawings were saved, to be opened only in the last month of 2014, after he requested a consultation. Now at the age of twenty-three, his major study was in Philosophy, but also wanted to be an artist with the use of computer techniques that he would be able to exploit for his own creative expression. He had a history of chronic cannabis use and was hospitalized for two weeks with a psychotic incident in September 2014. After his discharge while on medication, he reintroduced himself as the boy from the drawings. Now the time had arrived that these drawings could be interpreted either to guide him as a patient, or to find out if the exploration of this material could be instrumental in his recovery. This book is dedicated also to him. After two visits he decided out of his own free will not to return.

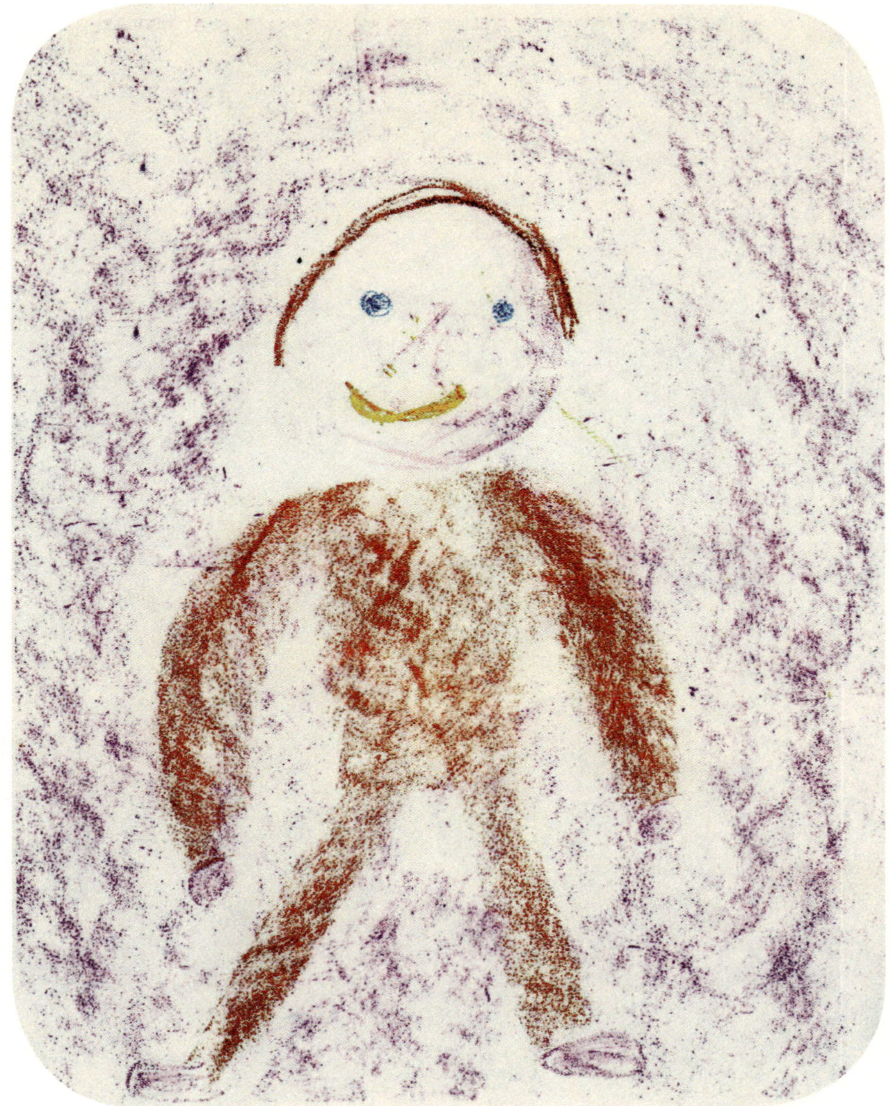

Plate 1: Standing boy

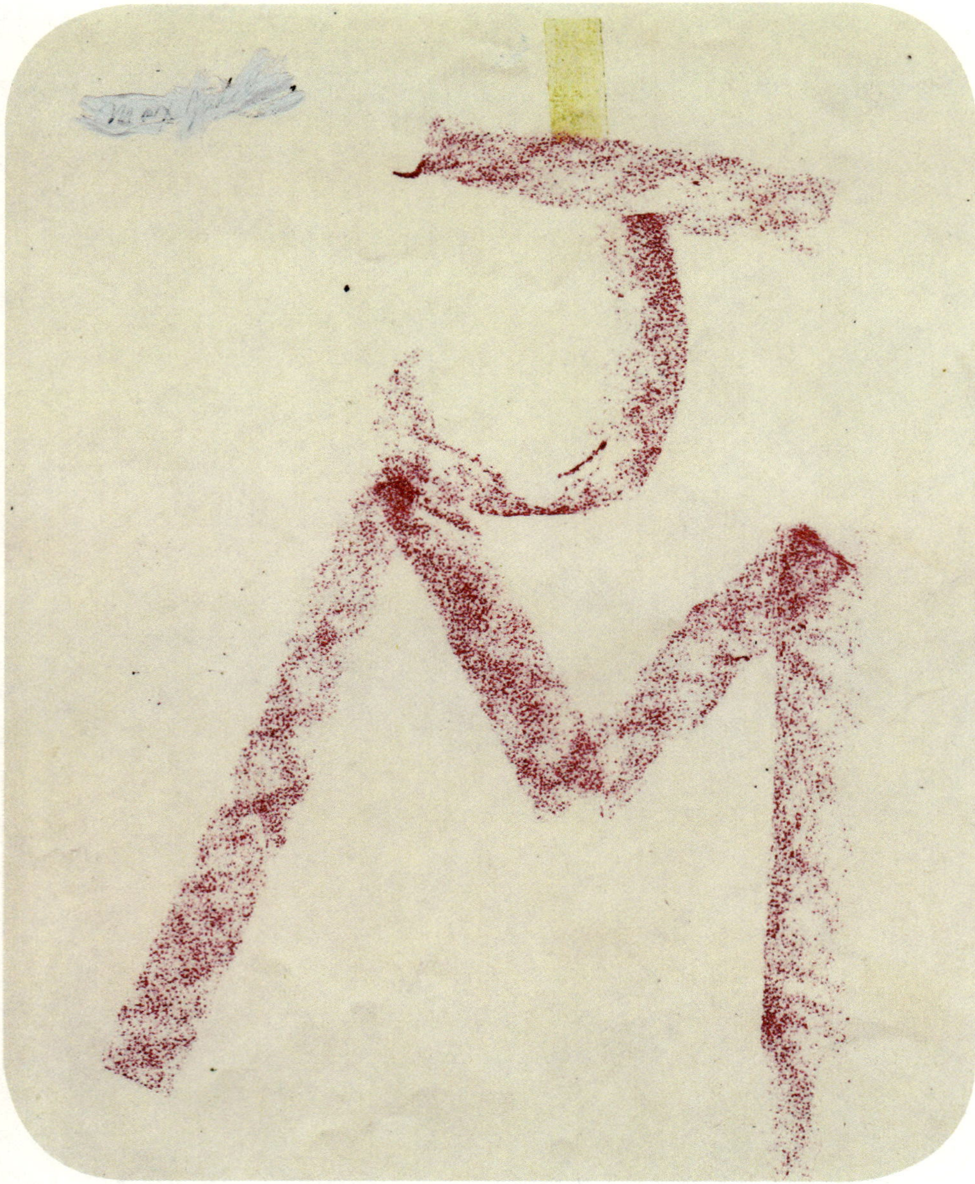

Plate 2: Signature as symbol

Asking the Child Artist for his "identification," Who are you? he presents me with a drawing (plate 1). For a six-year-old child, this is a complete representation of a person with hands and feet. The expression on the child's face is priceless and looking at the mature person now we can see a resemblance. Observe the courage and friendliness in this boy. Obviously this oil crayon drawing is a spontaneous result after a request and was finished within a few minutes.

After this drawing, he placed his "signature" in symbols on another page (plate 2). These consonants do not represent his real name, but must be reflecting a memory of a past identity or symbology.

Plate 3 (facing) is the first drawing the Child Artist represented to the team of observers. As is custom, using the house-tree-person assignment for the child, we learn about the capacity for balance and the innate connection the child has with its sources of light and warmth. (*For further explanation of this method in diagnostic evaluation we refer you to Audrey McAllen's work.*)

In the timespan the work of the class was handed in, we had no opportunity to examine and discuss the twenty children in the class. Only later, the outstanding figure of our Child Artist was noticed. The significance of this presentation was not fathomed at this time, but we all agreed that no questions or interrogation around his creation would be called for. And the question lingered in my mind, does this young being really know what he is drawing? Is he representing out of a conscious memory? Or, are his symbols a language he utilizes to make contact with a horizontal plane, meaning friends, teacher, and his own surroundings?

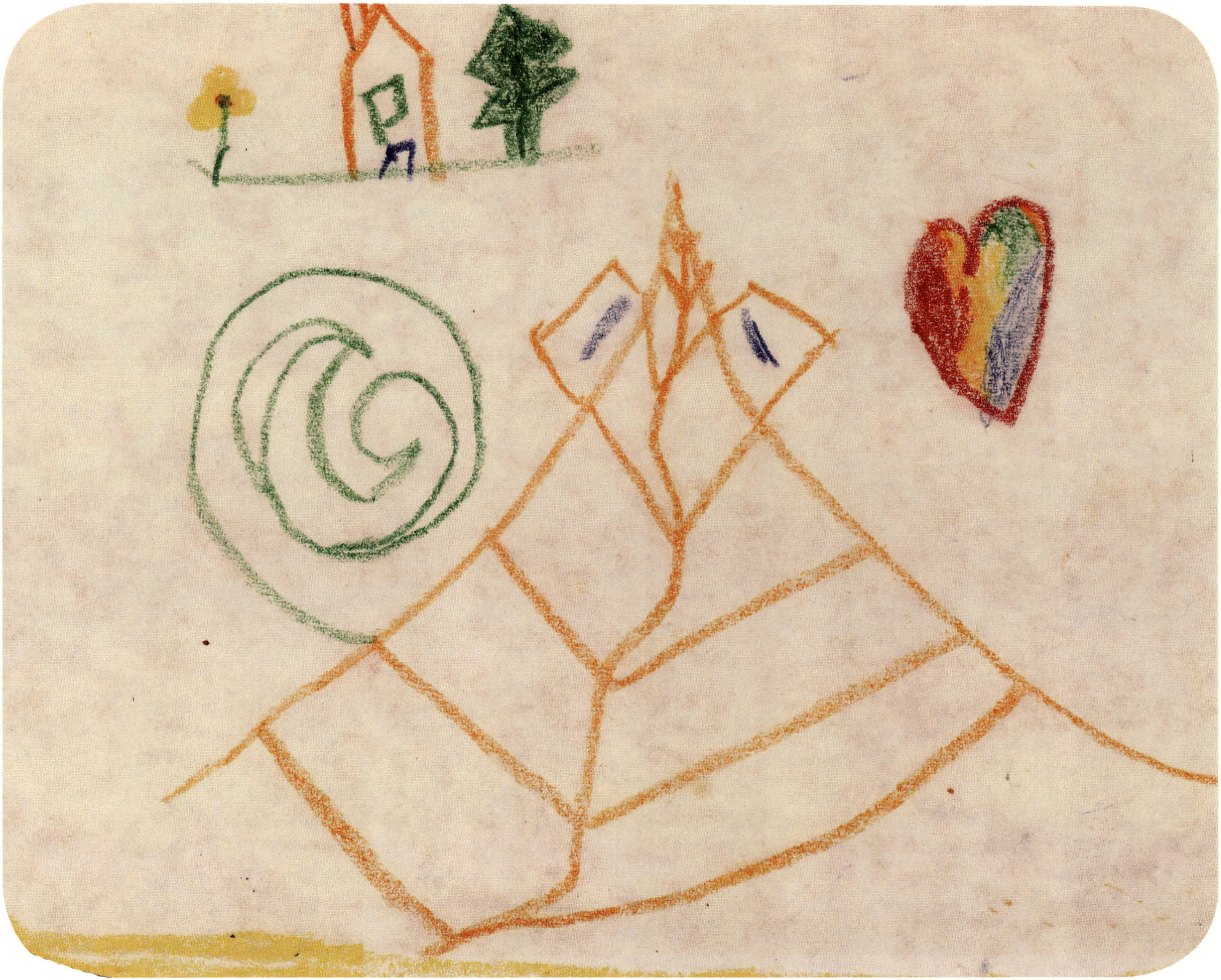

Plate 3: House, tree, person

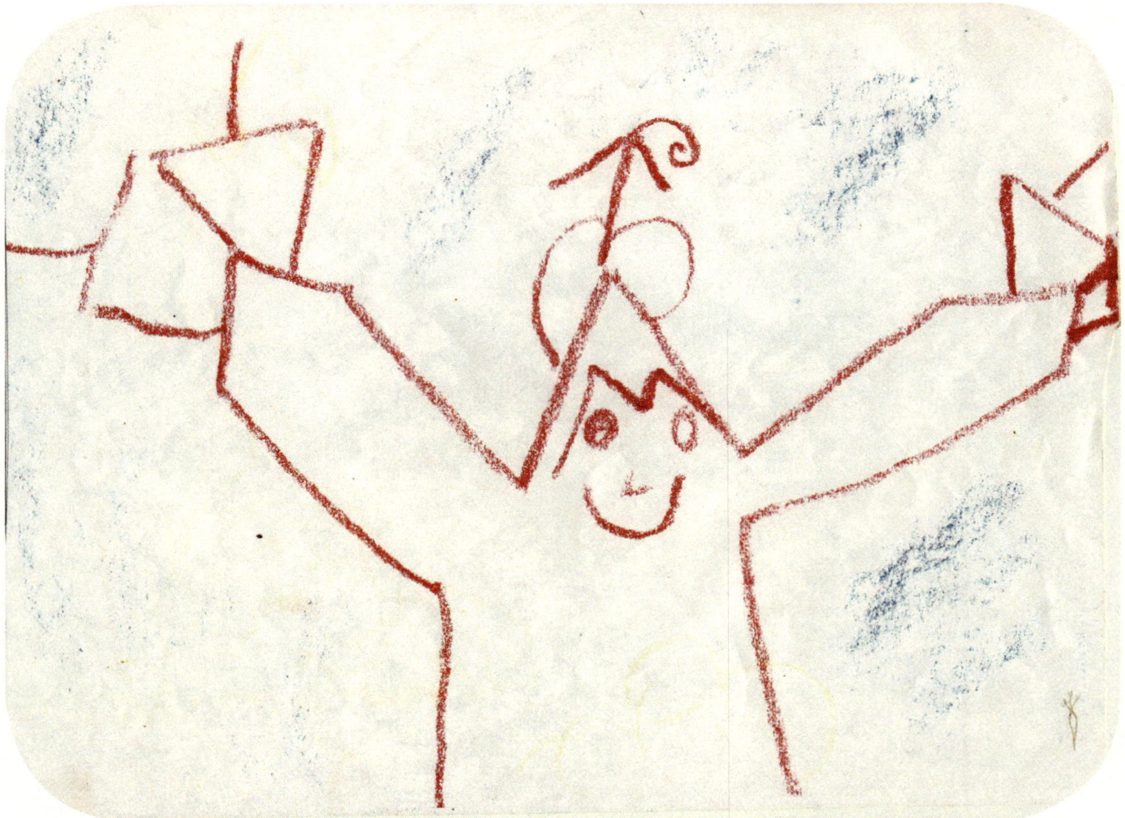

Plate 4: The Hierophant

His assignment is completed as a small vignette at the top of the paper. The house with a chimney window and door reflect a soul balance. The tree indicating his etheric force shows adequate leaf growth. He draws the person not as a human (which we later discovered he definitely could do), but as a flower. This pupil sees himself as a representative of the plant world. Attention is drawn to the figure in the center of the drawing. It represents a tent-like appearance complete with two extrusions or chimneys, one on each side of the pinnacle. There are seven pairs of ribs and a clear division between the right and the left side. On the right side of the dominating tent figure the Child Artist draws a spiral-like appendix to the tent. It is attached to the sixth rib, and at first interpretation we recognize an embryonic shape.

Detached from all of this, on the left side he draws a small heart-shaped form hanging in space, separate as an adornment. Here he uses the color red, blue, and green, a combination that is absent before. And in the middle of the heart we find a yellow winged figure. The same yellow as with the flower is used. Only with an enlargement of this detail the exquisite angelic being becomes prominent.

At our next visit to the school I took the opportunity to meet with the Child Artist again, just to really "meet" him and become better acquainted. It was obvious that I liked his picture very much. I asked if he could make me understand the dominating tent-like figure better, and within a few movements he handed me the picture of this extraordinary character.

The friendly face is capped by a pointed miter that reaches down between the eyes. It fits the microcephalic head structure tightly. The head is not rounded, but carries a heart-shaped, rounded protection from which an arrow-like protrusion reaches toward the heavens.

The fun part is the little curly tail that gives an impression of movement. There is no neck in this humanoid figure and arms are raised with two trapezoid surfaces on the end. Each of these organs is equipped with a hair or antenna. The right protrusion represents a pointed structure giving room to two trapezoid surfaces, each with an antenna repeated on the left side. There is no ambivalence here! It really is not important what I think these pictures show. It is the viewer who develops an imagination as to what such a symbol could represent.

The story of the Child Artist and me becomes more personalized. At the time of our visits, he carefully listened to my request. Of course I could not help being curious about where the pictures would lead me. By now I was certain that I could learn something that he could convey only through his artistic talent. For the adult, it becomes a symbolic language that associates past disciplines with hidden inner experiences and interpretations. I refrain from interpreting what he shows me as an alien being. This time I want further clarification of the humanoid figure he gave me earlier. Indeed, he can now lead me into the world of alchemical contraptions used in ancient laboratories.

The structure in plate 5 is shaped like a house with four doors on the ground floor. The middle area of this imaginative device provides the viewer with a large window (looking in or out?) and two arms that could be chimneys, which also have small windows. The top level has a separate, blue window. Is this individuality using distinct colors to indicate different functions? I have seen this "oven" before; it is an alchemical *Athanor,* or furnace. The bottom contains the oven fire. In the middle region the water baths are suspended over the fire. Above this. steam escapes, and adjacent to it an apparatus for distillation is incorporated. The flue area in the attic provides a breathing capacity for the whole. The bell-shaped contraption I cannot explain.

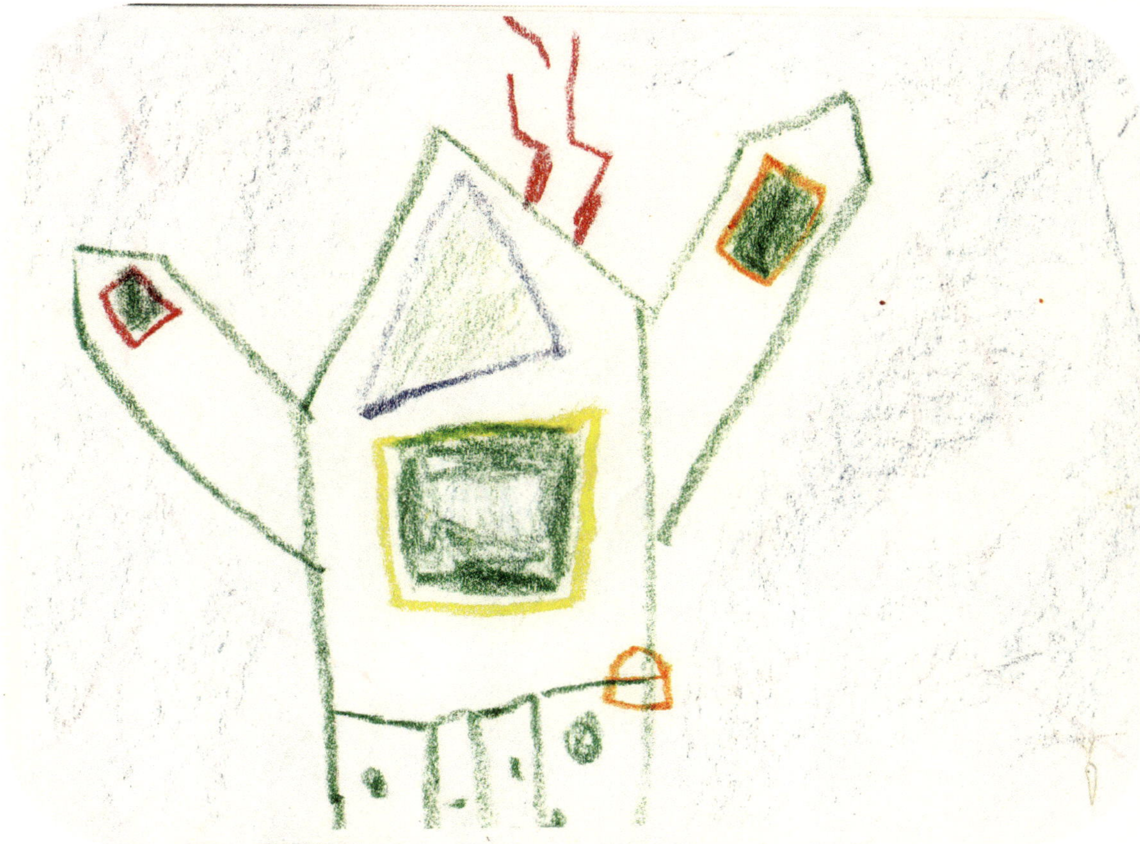

Plate 5: Metamorphosis of hierophant to house

The opulent home with two fireplaces and chimneys is executed by another pupil. No symbolic language is recognized, where with the drawing of the Child Artist the viewer is stirred with memories of the Athanor.

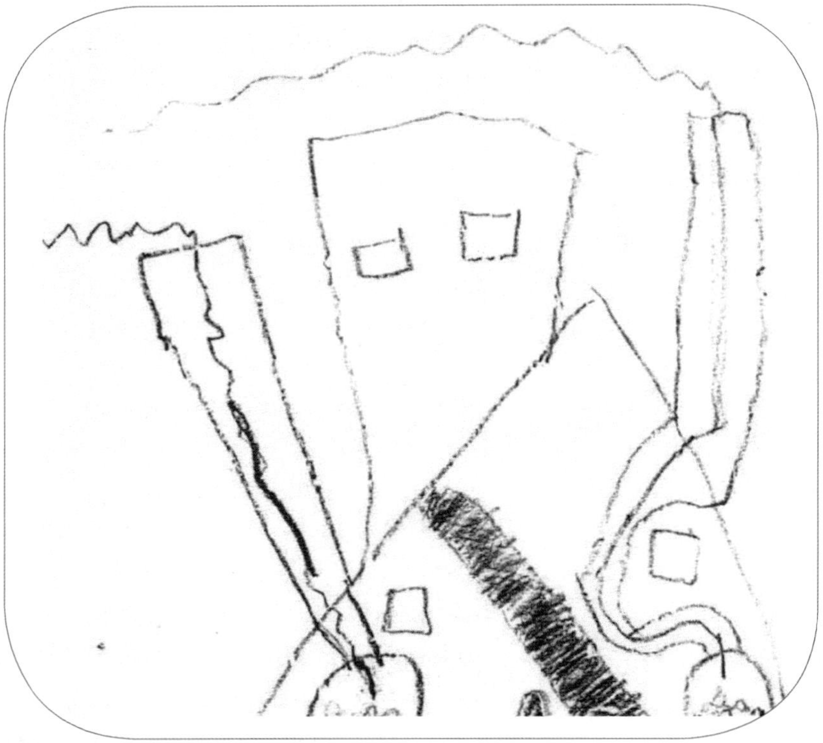

Plate 6: Comparative drawing of home

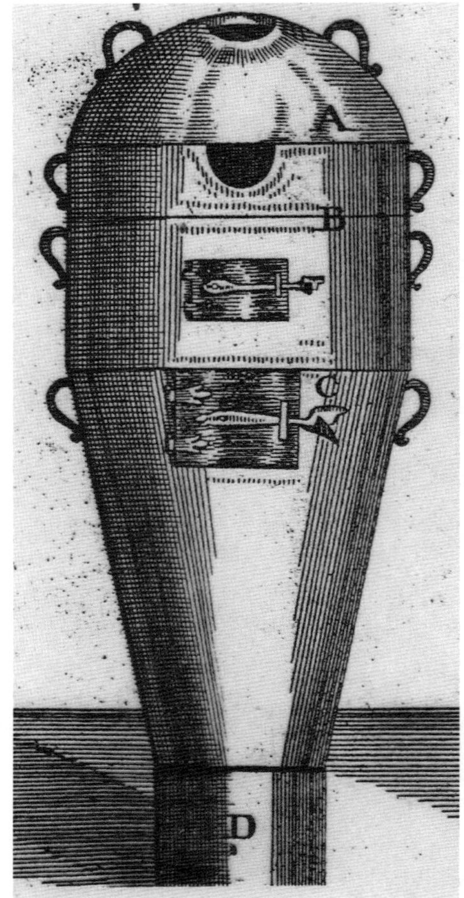

Plate 7: Alchemical Oven. Used in chemical laboratories, this was an oven in which the complicated chemical processes of evaporation, distillation, condensation, and calcination were observed through a window, enabling the chemist to apply full control (refer to Museum Collections by Alexander Roob).

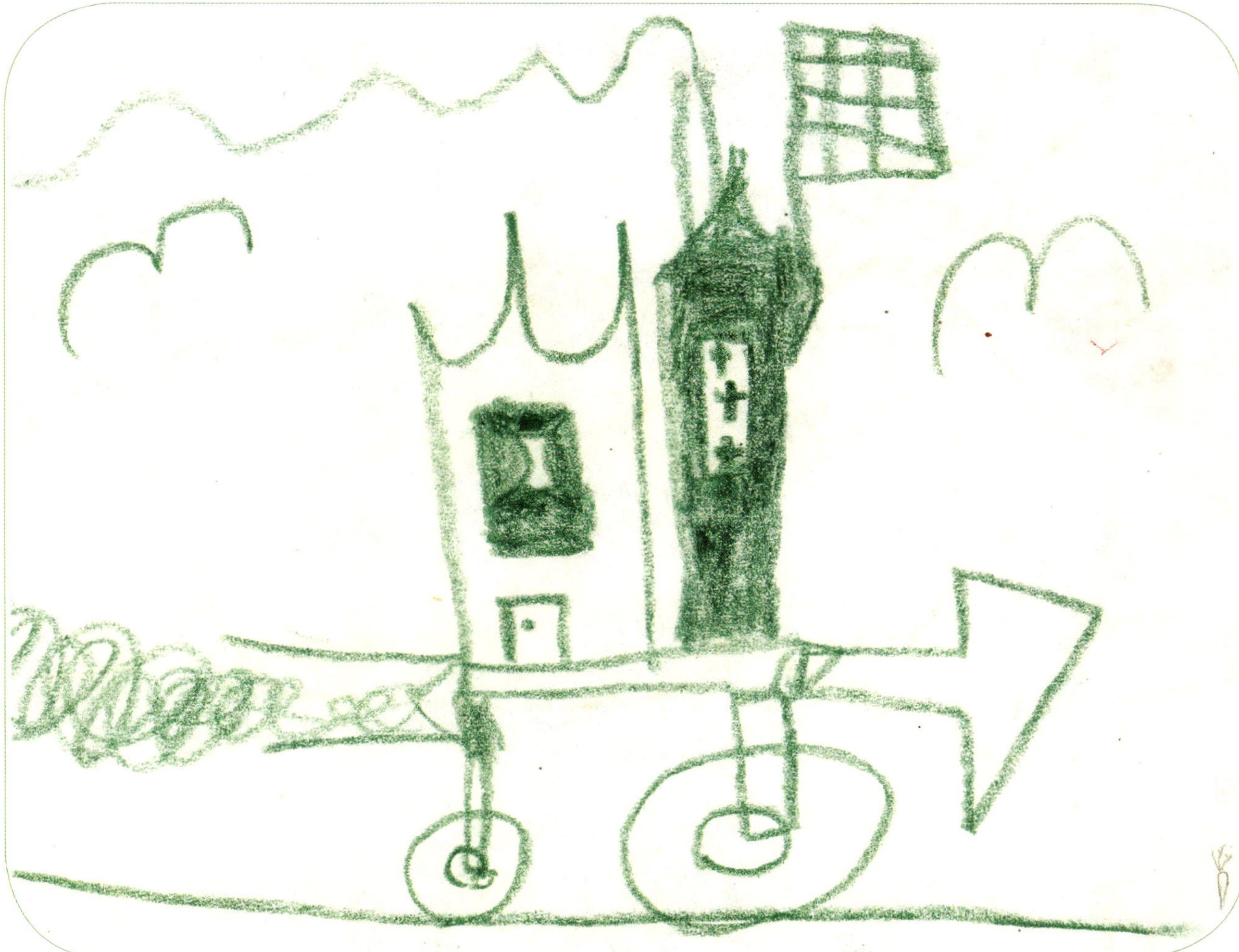

Plate 8: The Green Truck

The Child Artist playfully introduces movement to me. When he draws a conveyance, inner joyfulness and ebullience are communicated. It is a four-wheel vehicle clearly moving from left to right; the arrow, seen as the front "bumper," clearly tells us the direction. The smoke coming from the back of the carriage expresses speed—I would say very fast—which is also evident in the smoke from the front section, which must be the engine. The flag is waving straight forward?

The comparison between motor and cabin is very obvious. The cabin has a door with an elaborate window and a crown-like roof top. The feminine is earmarked as royalty. Merging of the male and female element gives rise to new life, expressed symbolically with the flying birds or the fountain symbol. This drawing has an uncanny likeness to what Roob represents as the chemical bi-gender representation (*refer plate A*).

What is different in plate 7 is the oven on the right represents the male element, where the potbellied or receptive retort (*cucurbit*) is placed next to it and referred to as the female element. The "Chymical Wedding" occurs both outwardly and inwardly.

Interpreting the final drawing from the Child Artist is for me the beginning of an exploration into the meaning of this exquisite gift he placed in my hands. As in the Gnostic myth, it involves a polarity. The Good and the Evil present themselves in their balanced capacity. Humanity meets the devouring monster and can slay it only after many painful sojourns into the depth of the Earth. On the horizontal plane, the domain of darkness, cacophony, and false gods, the overpowering jaws can annihilate me. It attacks my life force; it comes to me in the guise of a huge head with ferocious teeth; its small triangular body is chaotic, and the limbs are rudimentary. Is this *me?* The question lingers: Who can be identified as the Child Artist? Still in our midst, how can he be met? Do we want to pave a way to better listening and understanding?

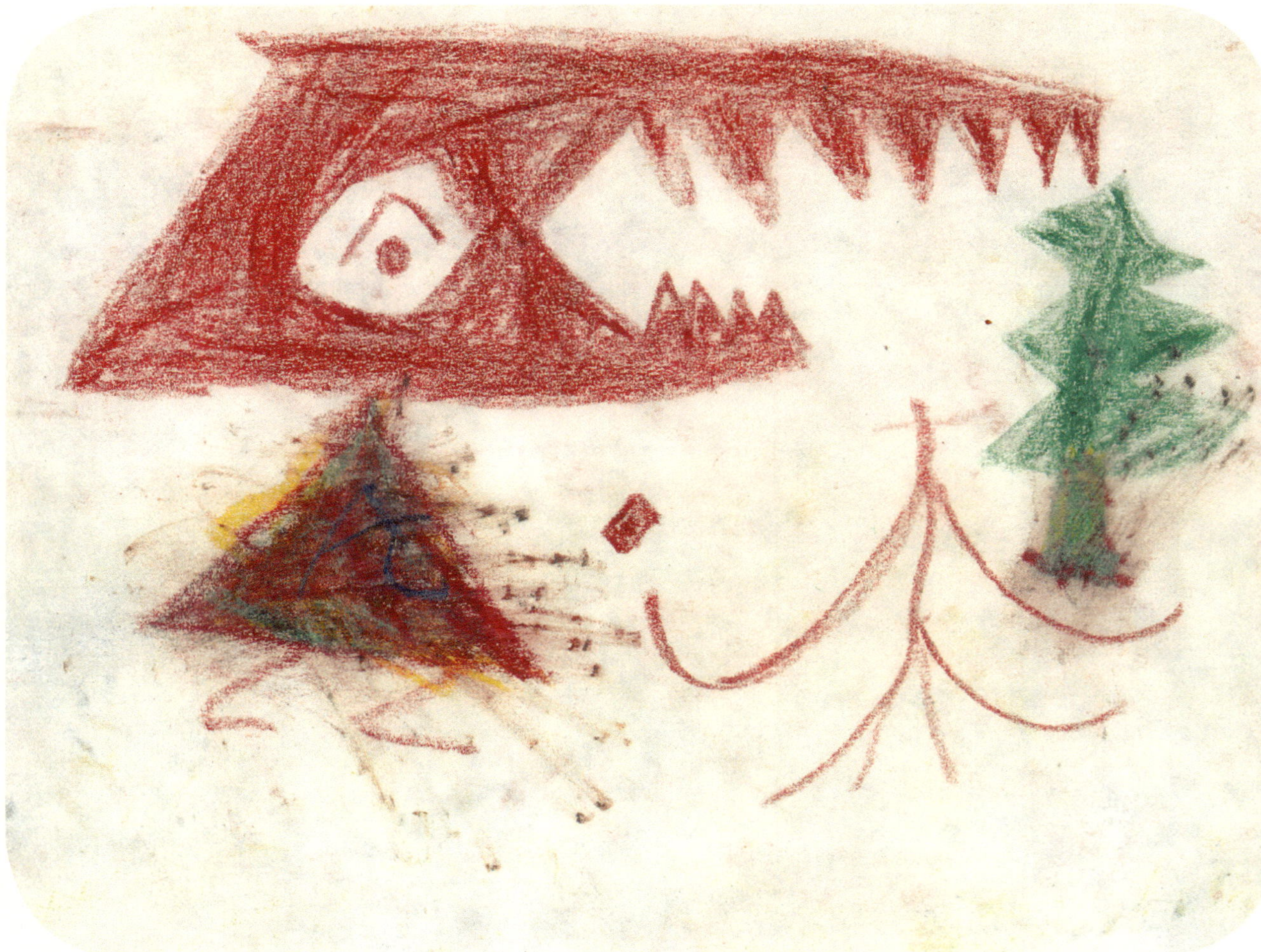

Plate 9: The Devouring Monster

The symbolic nature of the work that the Child Artist shared with me has become very clear. Some of the symbols are frequently drawn in the sketches. I want to further examine and identify three of them with the genius behind these simple expressions.

Process of Consolidation

In plate 10 we see a spiral, and only the color red is used. He starts the figure from the periphery and slowly wends his way inward, meticulous with balance and conforming to the space of the paper. He repeats the journey inward six times, with only one correction in the first circle. To complete the balance, he orients the spiral by "grounding" it with an anchor, or feet, but does not forget antennae for the upper region. The Child Artist points to:

1) the idea of the spiral for condensing forces;
2) the anchor to illustrate gravity of the Earth;
3) the antennae to acknowledge the presence of imponderable force from above.

The expression of creation as a flow from phase to new phase until the final solid state becomes a reality is represented sublimely in this spiral. The Spiritual Science of Rudolf Steiner introduces genesis in warmth, light, air, water, life-chemistry, and atom. I have taken this sketch as an example of the final solid state, earth, in the genesis sequence of creation (R. Steiner, *Occult History*).

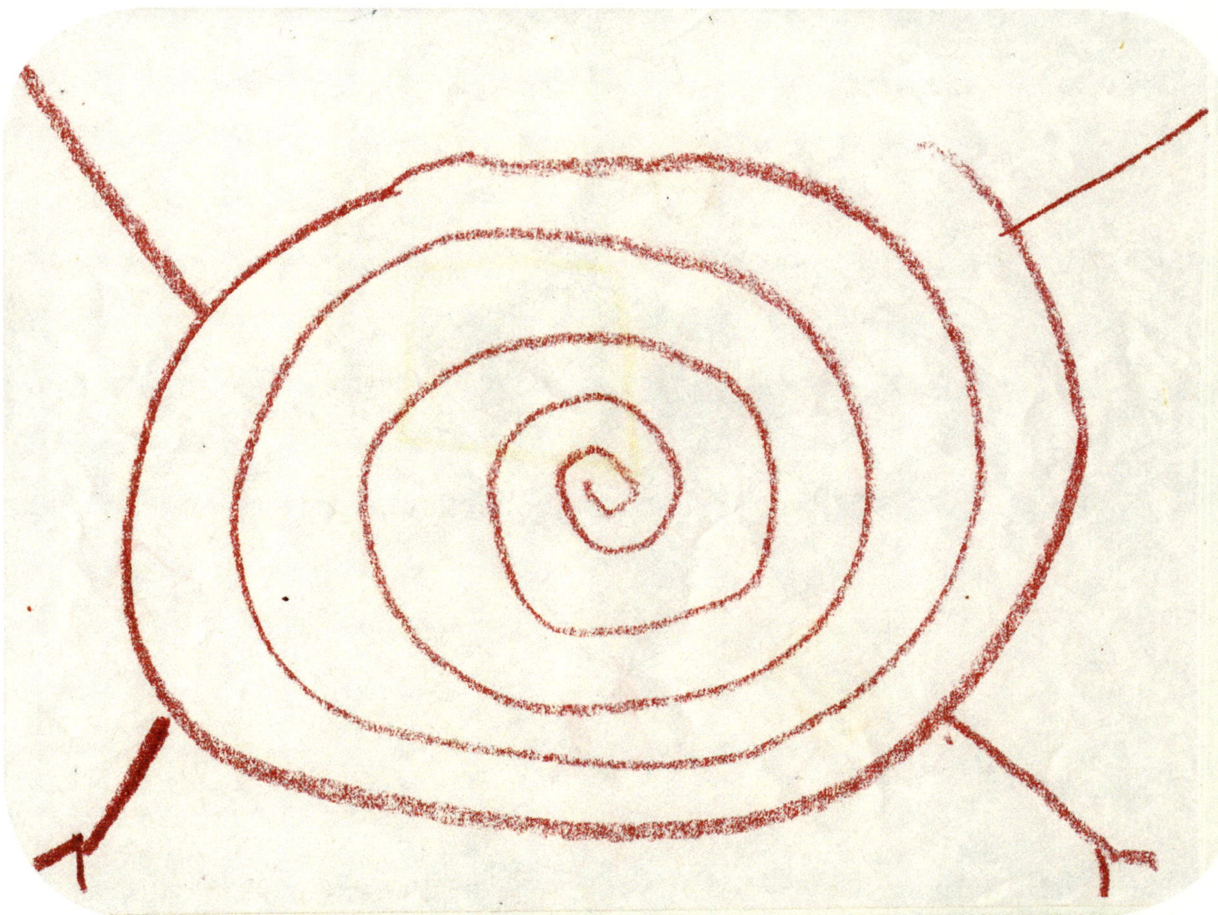

Plate 10: Process of consolidation

DROP-formation

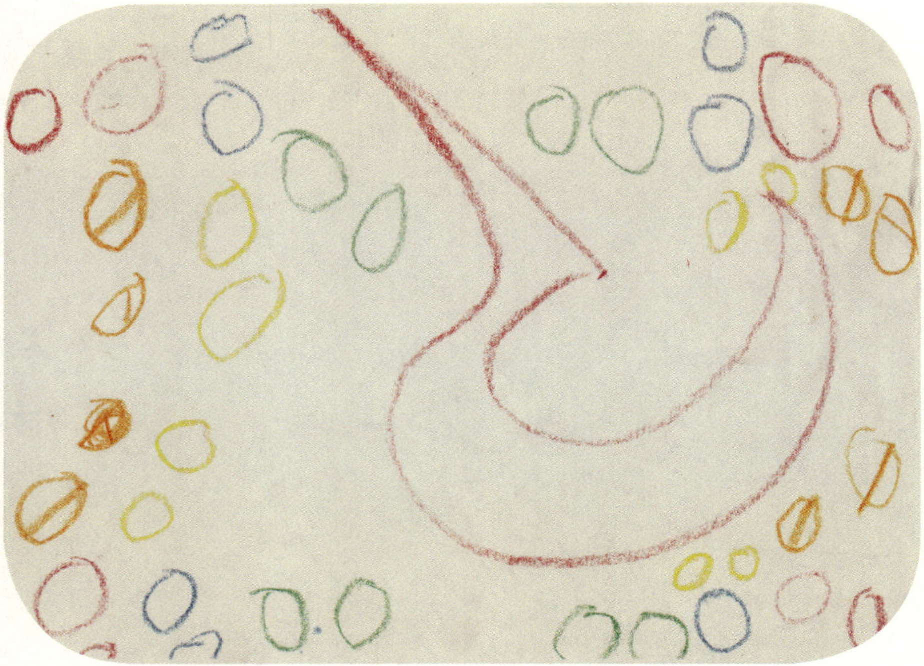

Plate 11a: Drop formation—pelican eggs

The centerpiece of this sketch is an exquisite figure that resembles a pelican. Turning the picture around it could also be interpreted as a sickle. Since we have no indication of the proper orientation, I would first like to use the analogy of the pelican likeness. This bird is used as an alchemical, or Hermetic, symbol and represents "she" who brings her dead young (the base metals) back to life with her own blood (tincture). Our Child Artist uses a display of colors for this picture to represent pairs of droplets—a multitude of them, with five pairs in each corner. Are these eggs? This picture reflects an inherent compulsive nature of the artist, both through the constancy of the five pair of circles in the four regions and the consistent choice of the colors green, blue, red, yellow, and brown. In the brown "egg" we find repeated shadowing.

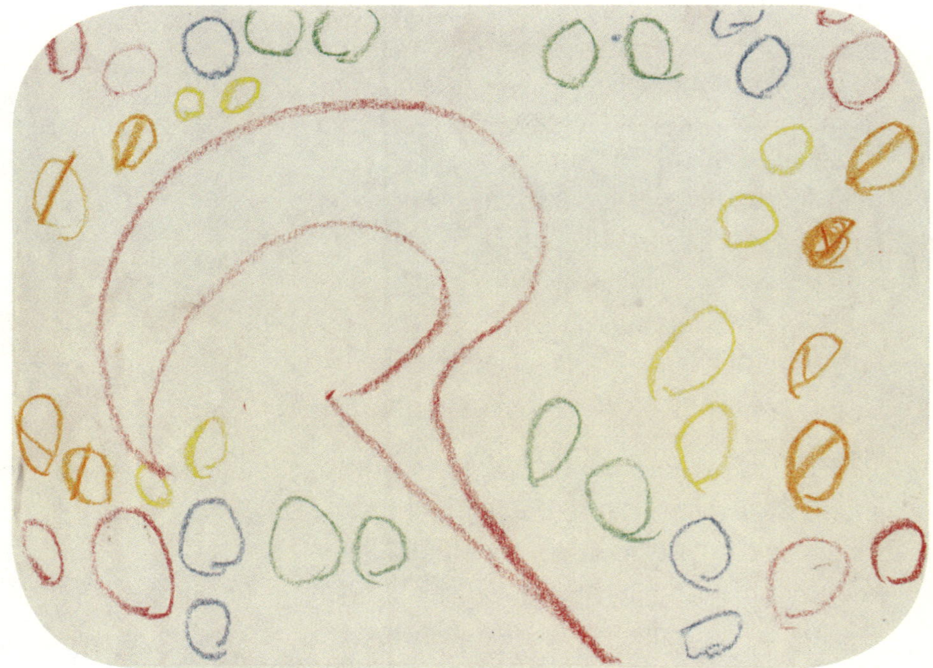

Plate 11b: Drop formation—sickle

Turning the sketch 180 degrees we come closer to the function of drop formation through the cleavage of streaming liquid. Referring to the early formative stage of the embryo, I also call this a mercurial process. The signature that typifies the liquid metal is droplet formation, atmospheric dispersion, and/or condensation. This heavy metal is unique in its characteristics and, in an imaginative way, can be likened to the blood, cell structure, and circulation.

The next sets of sketches need to be combined into a series (plates 12, 13, 14). Close examination reveals the journey that the Child Artist has to undertake to come to rest in the "grail" prepared for him on Earth.

In plate 12, we see the first stage in which the Cosmic Chariot has left the "heavenly" home. The symbol for Sun and Moon are on the left, indicating that he is a child from our universe. The cosmic sail is magnificent, perfectly rounded with intricate wiring connected to a rudder. The arrows indicate where the boat will go—away from there to here. On the front bow, connected to a platform or rope-like structure, we observe an amorphous figure that is definitely part of the overall presentation. The cabin is closed. We get a sense that a passive exchange is enacted between passenger and vehicle. The rudder will be discussed in future detail.

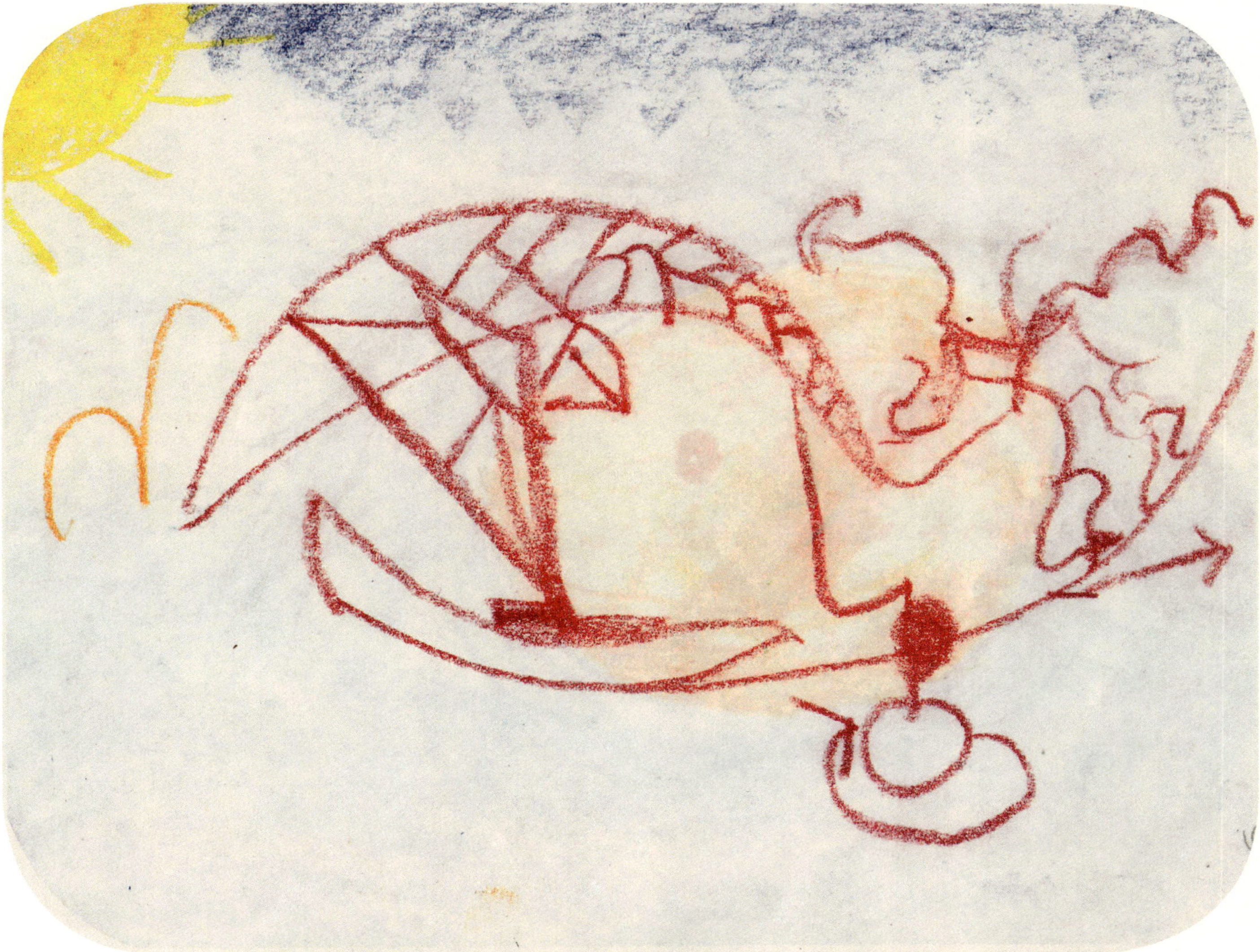

Plate 12: Departure from Sun region

Plate 13 is truly one of the most enthralling sketches by the Child Artist, reflecting his genius in involving the viewer with his enthusiasm, his control over his vehicle, and the independence he now can assert. As in the representation of the Three Kings, here, too, we are witnessing movement. The waters are choppy; he is definitely "going down" but in full control, sitting high and dry in a throne-like chair, and handling the way down to his destiny. The sled has no sail, and we sense that the vehicle has become an extension of his own image, a chariot fit for a king. Most prominent is the rudder-like protrusion in the aft, bearing a distinct resemblance to the previous rudder image.

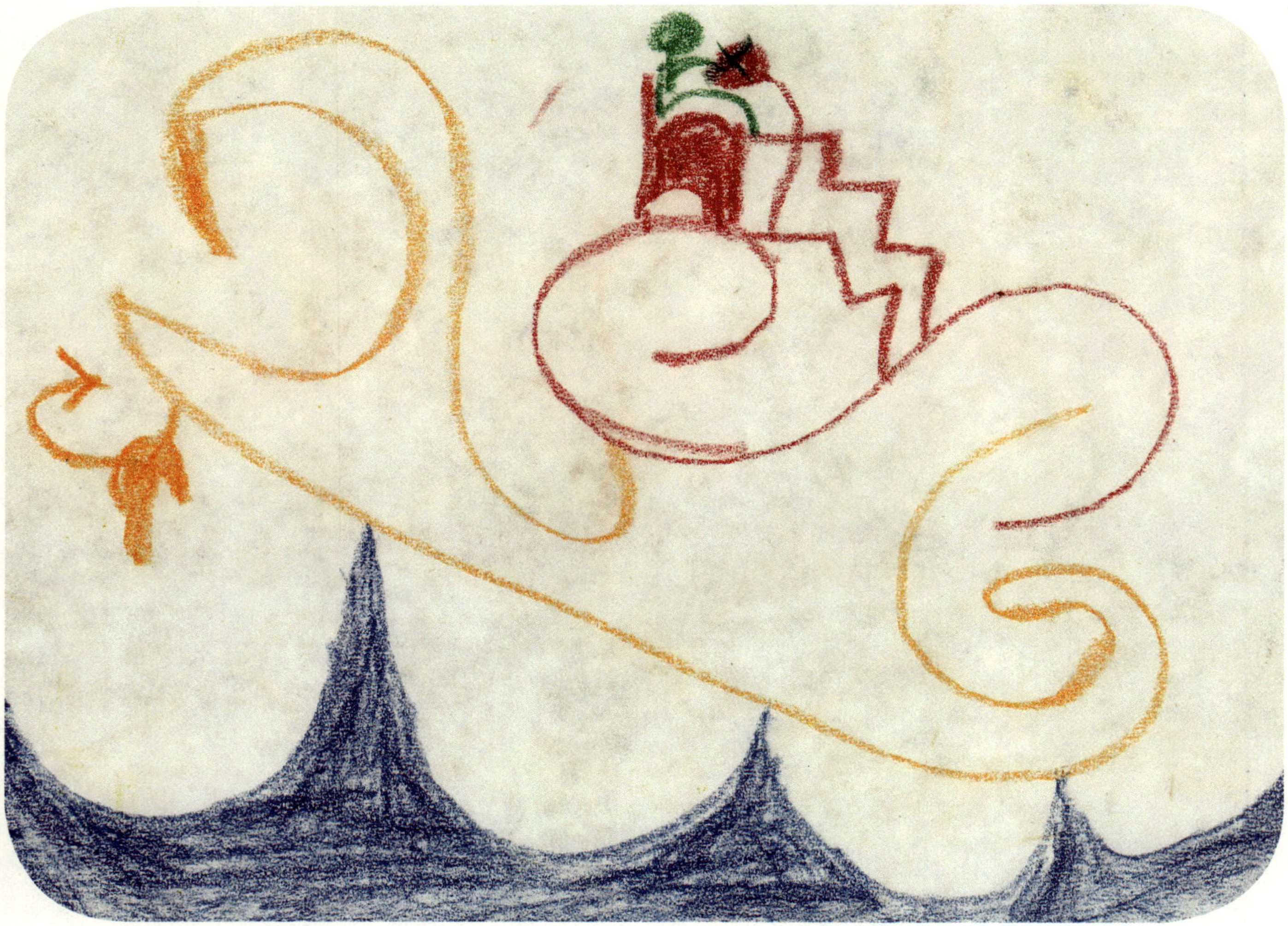

Plate 13: Cosmic sled in choppy waters

With plate 14, the final moment has arrived. The traveler has left the ship with wing-shaped sails still fully deployed. Could he return? Earthly phenomena surround the intimidated little man—symbols of hearts, fountains, and something resembling earphones. The most important being overshadowing the figure—and in fact the whole picture is a large shadowy humanoid presence with a very long arm that surrounds the little child protectively. No, he is not alone. A guide will be with him to ensure his incarnation as a human citizen. The earphones are an indication that he will become deaf to the music of the spheres. The realization that silence from the cosmic spheres will become a reality hangs as a dominant presence over the sketch. He can establish himself on Earth only by the life force (yellow underneath the boat) supporting his heart forces. Both guardian and the young traveler look toward the right, the blue yonder as the destiny of their travels.

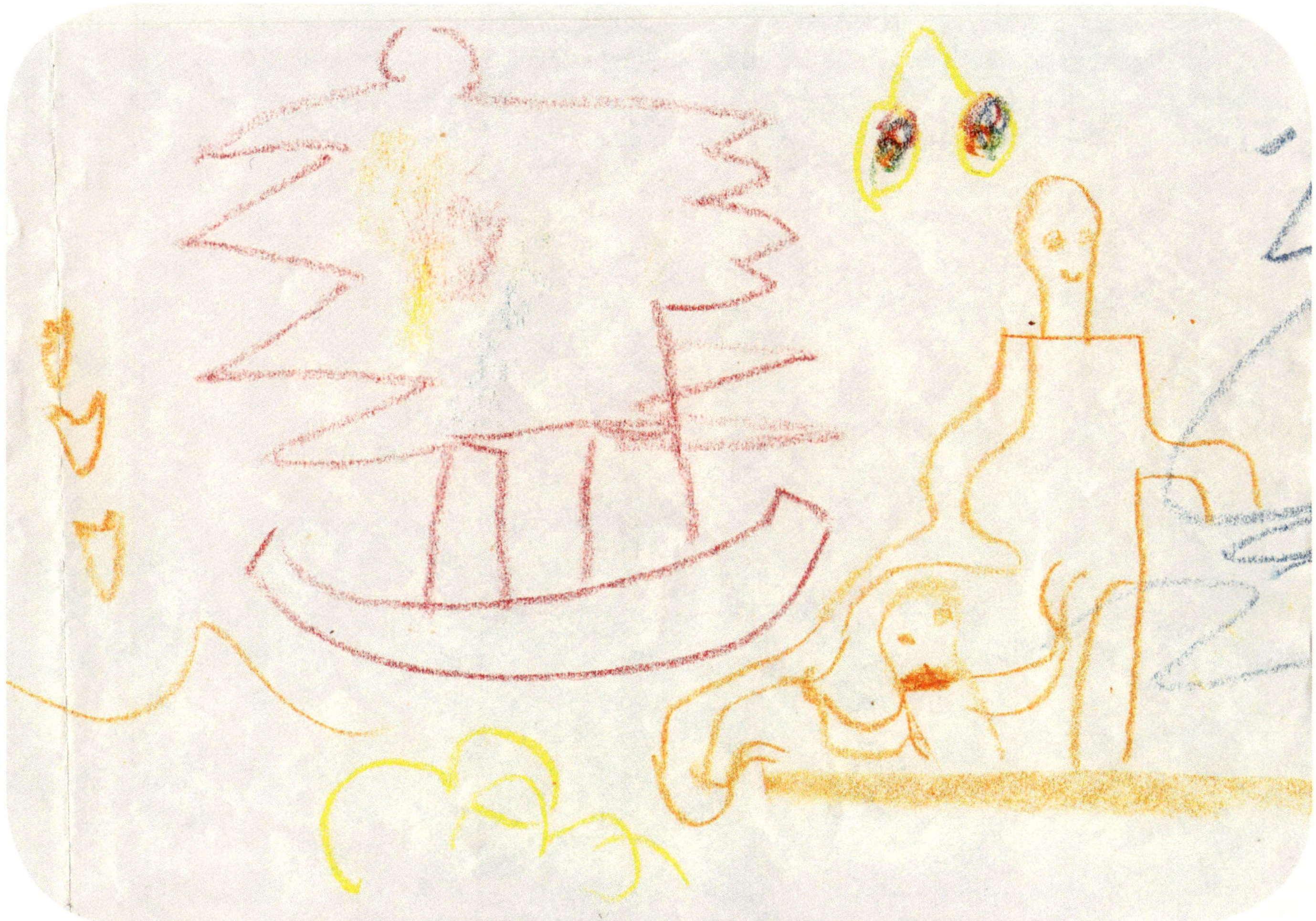

Plate 14: On Earth—end of journey

This magnificent multi-colored sketch, plate 15, has become the central illustration for all the steps we will examine in describing the embryonic development. The interesting aspect of this drawing is the two-time division into a threefold organization of the human embryo. First the Child Artist is capable of reminding the viewer of the threefold constitution of mineral, plant, and animal kingdoms represented in the human embryo. Second, he reveals in the center the threefold organization we find when the embryo divides into the three structures of ectoderm, mesoderm, and endoderm. The three body parts clearly indicated to be the upper region as central nervous system, the middle realm with heart–lung (prominently the vertebral "anlage"), and in the lower pole a representation of liver under the diaphragm. It could also be seen as an embryonic form; the viewer is free to interpret it subjectively.

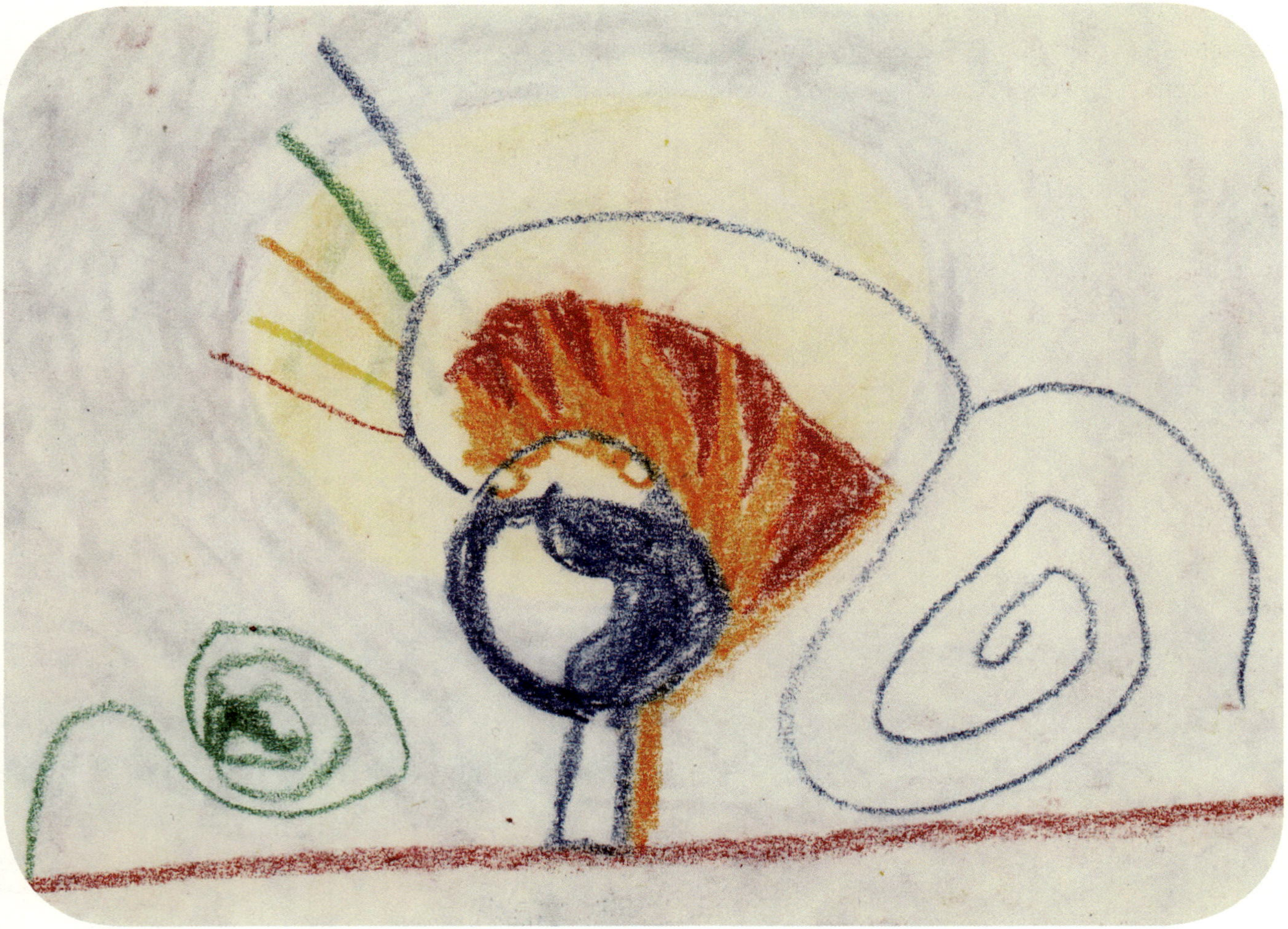

Plate 15: Template for embryogenesis

This sketch has been fragmented, enlarged, and made to fit many descriptions of embryo development. The method is scientifically questionable, yet inspiration from his work, as well as a sense of wonder, accompanies me throughout the study of this Child Artist's efforts to convey a message to humanity. What is the message and can we hear? Does the message refer to the steps of the Emerald Tablet?

The Child Artist draws a similar structure for us three times. It is significant enough to reproduce here as a fragment from the larger representation. All three figures consist of a connecting rod, a round heart-shaped body, and an arrow protrusion. The round body connects directly with the main frame. For the moving objects, the curled arrow points toward the destination of the vehicle. In plate 3, the arrow points to the region above.

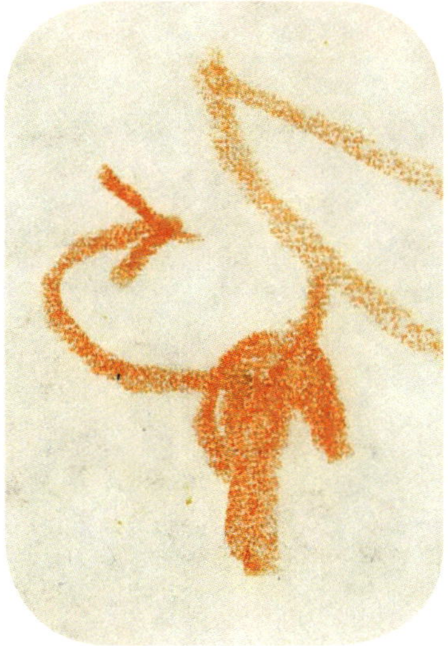

Plate 16a: The Rudder (fragment a)

The arrow in the three drawings could have an esoteric significance; it becomes a symbol that the viewer can apprehend while studying the sketches in depth.

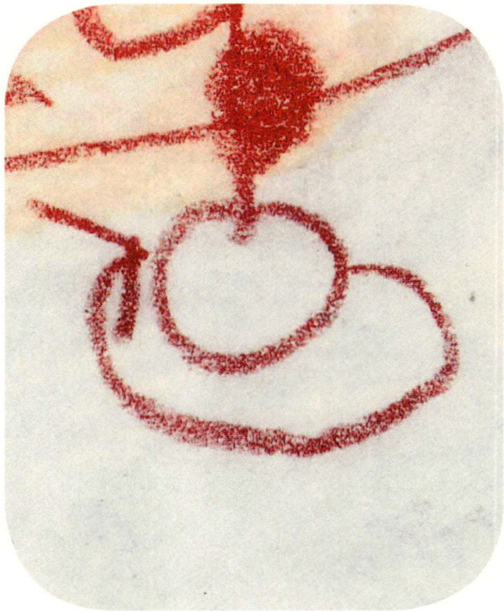

Plate 16b: The Rudder (fragment b)

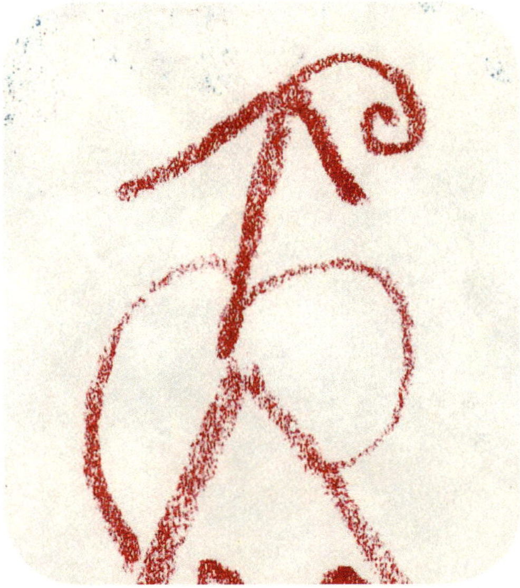

Plate 16c: The Rudder—headpiece of the hierophant

Gesture of Dispersion

The symbol for life is displayed prominently in many of these drawings: a spring coming from the earth with gushing water; the many symbols of bird-like silhouettes all indicate this creative process. Moreover, the Moon is related closely to the watery element—not in a literal sense, of course, but in the hermetic vocabulary the Moon sphere equates with the feminine, fecundity the living water, and the fountain of youth.

I have an imagination that a process of dispersal is presented with this "fountain." From the state of solidity, transformation to a gaseous state is an essential metamorphosis in alchemical work. The Child Artist understood the concept of polarities, or processes in nature that have contrasting effects. I will explore this further in the text on Alchemy.

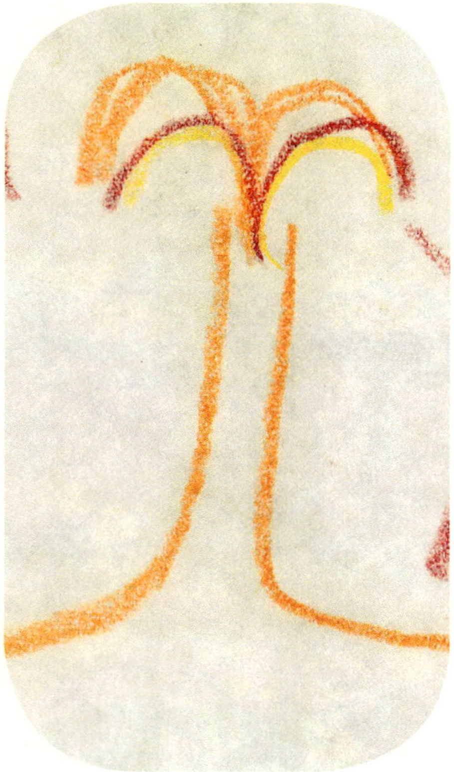

Plate 17a: Dispersion—artesian

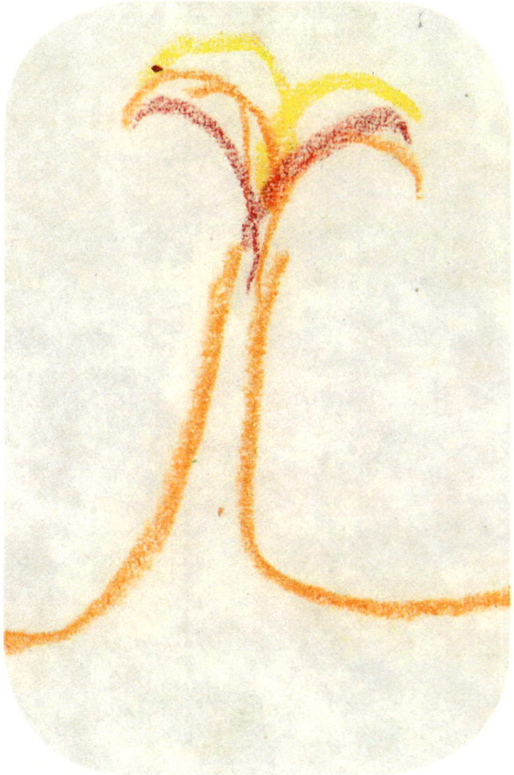

Plate 17b: Dispersion—fountain

Gesture of Consolidation

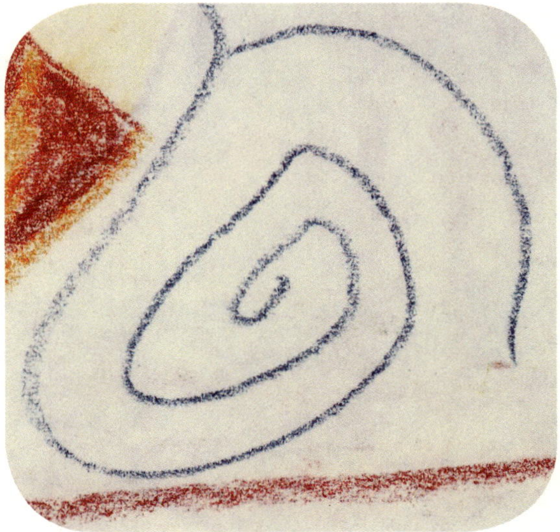

Plate 18: Gesture of consolidation

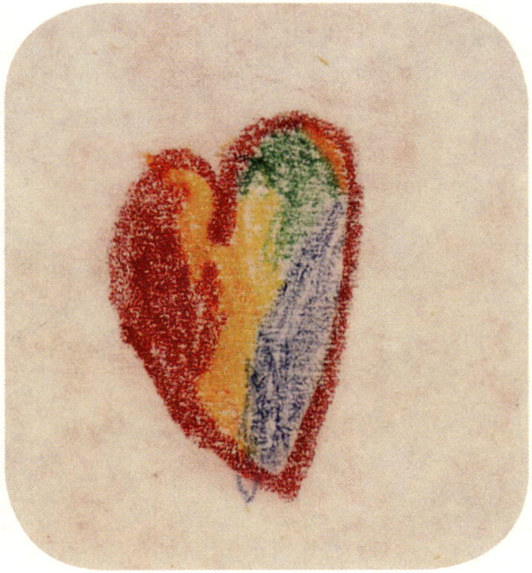

Plate 20a: Heart (fragment)

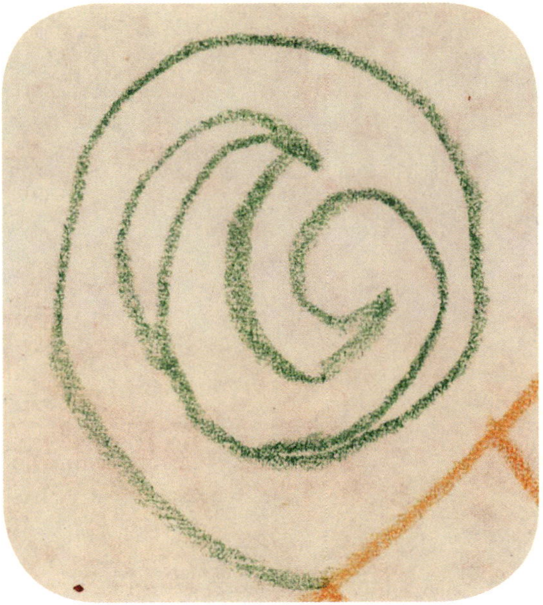

Plate 19: Consolidation—embryo

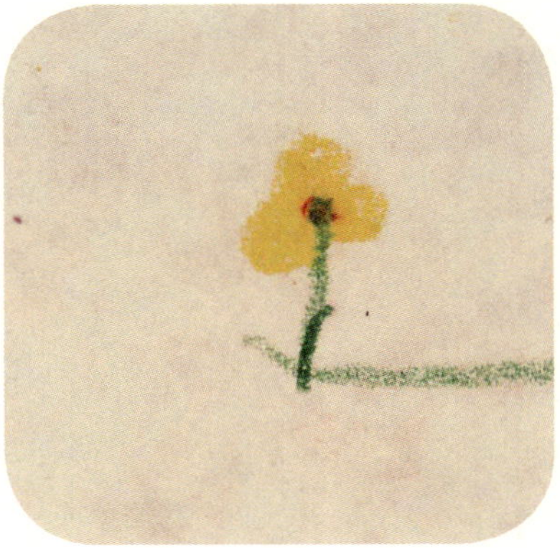

Plate 20b: Flower (fragment)

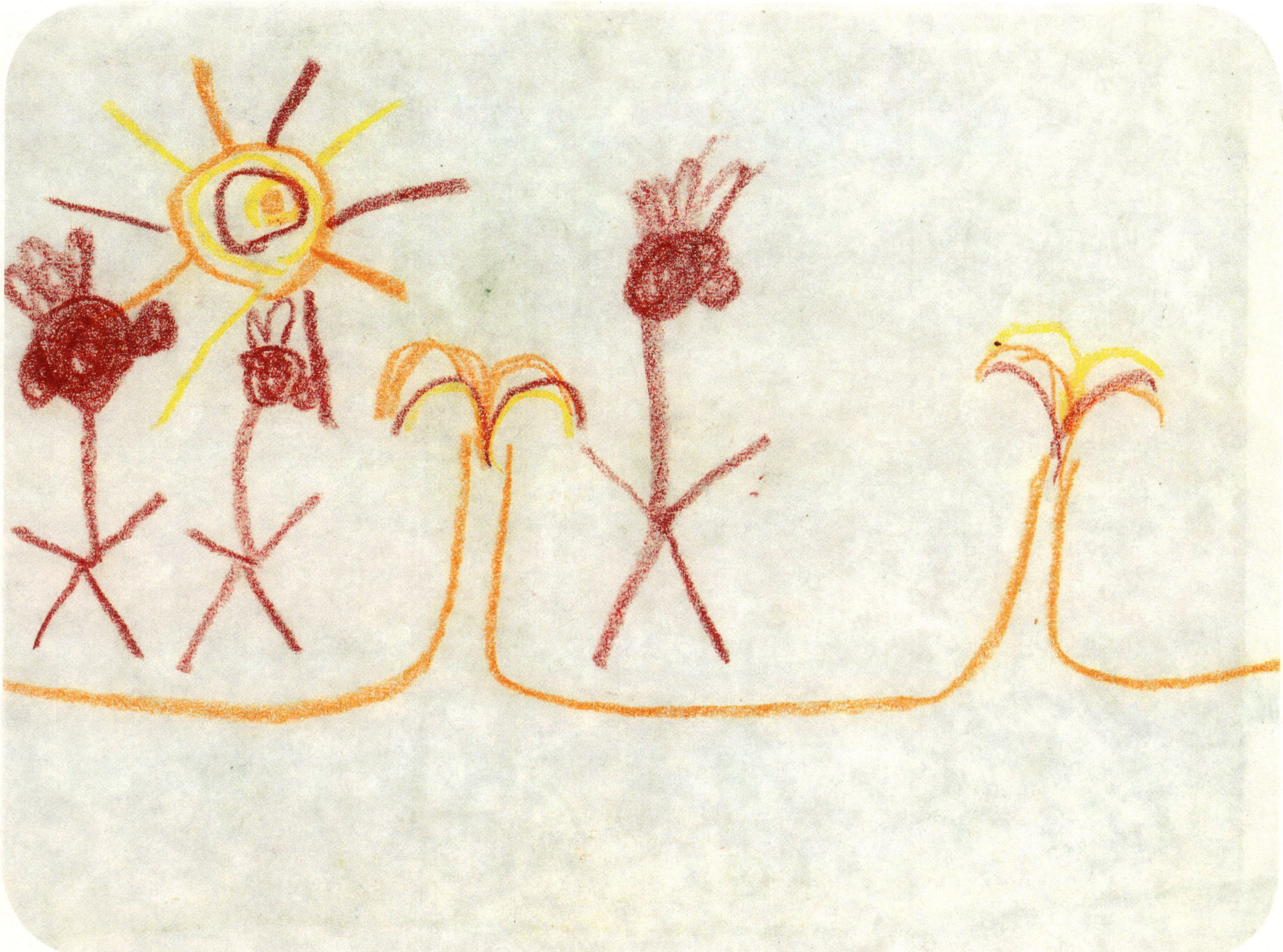

Plate 21: *The initiation of kings*

The Initiation of Kings

The figures of the Three Kings were the Child Artist's greatest gift to me and were instrumental in opening my world toward writing down the experiences I had to undergo with the evaluation of his sketches. For years these pictures had been stashed away while I did not know how to interpret this valuable elegant material. A health-crisis sixteen years after his sharing set the wheel of action in motion. The question was if, in my role as a physician, the wonders of his gift after exploration could help to restore his inner balance. Did he need a verification of the existence of the vertical infinite world filled with spirit?

Let is carefully examine this landscape sketch, which is executed in three colors red, orange, and yellow. What immediately strikes me is that the picture seems to move, meaning that the figures, each one wearing a crown, are moving from the left to the right. They are experiencing some kind of ceremony that I need to identify. Two sources of "energy" or forces are present. In the upper left we see the Sun, but with careful examination one can identify a being in the center. I feel comfortable to name this source the radiant giver of warmth and light. Undoubtedly, this living being becomes a part of the initiation. The other source of life comes from below, from the Earth, so to say. Here the living water bursts forth out of the center of the Earth. The figures are initiated one by one in a moving order from left to right. The Sun bestows the life, as we know it on Earth, in the gift of warmth and light. The Earth sustains the life with water and her solidity. Together they become the Living Water of the organism imbued with life.

So who are these Kings? Literally are there three initiated figures or am I being introduced to the "Thrice Blessed King" also introduced as Hermes Trismegistus? Let us examine this further.

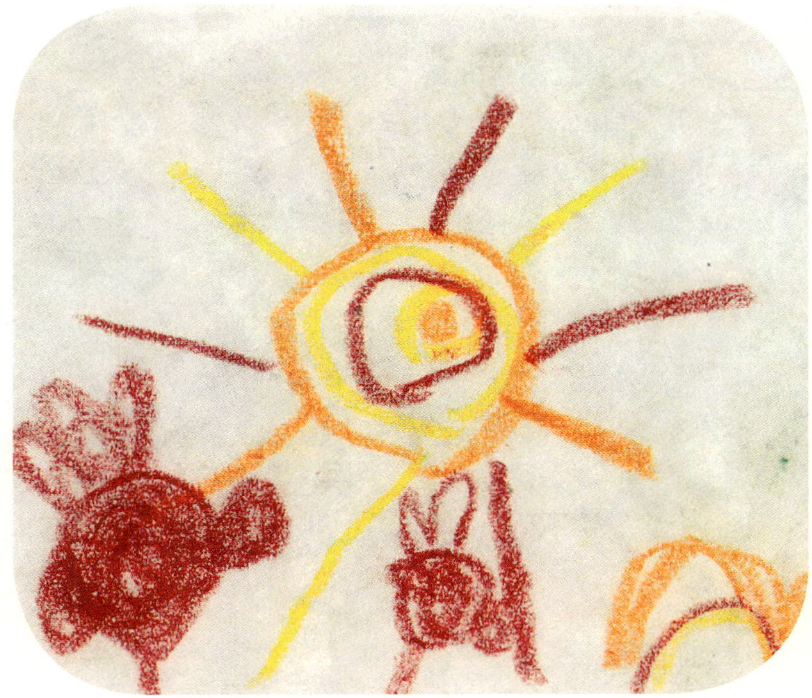

Plate 22: Sun (fragment)

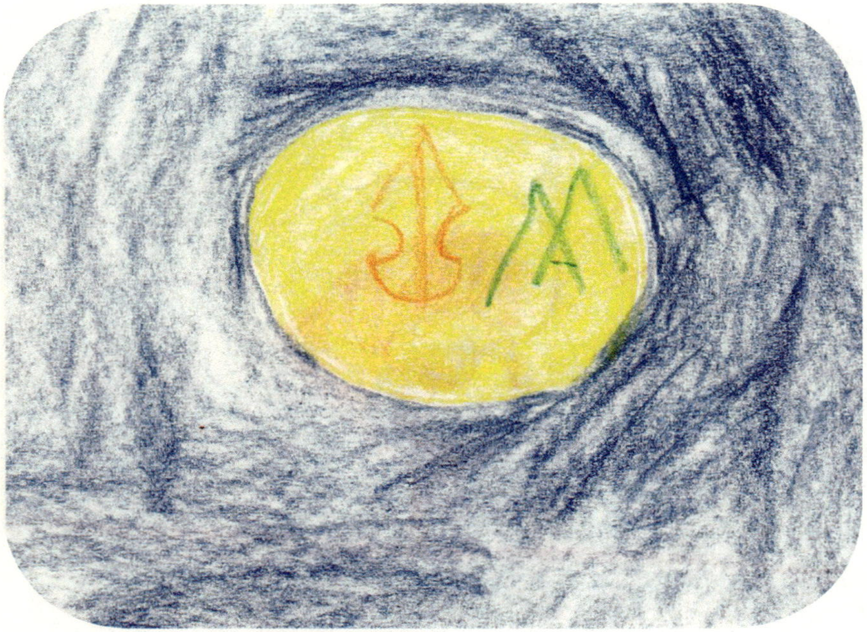

Plate 23: Symbols in the Sun

Plate 24: Face of the Moon

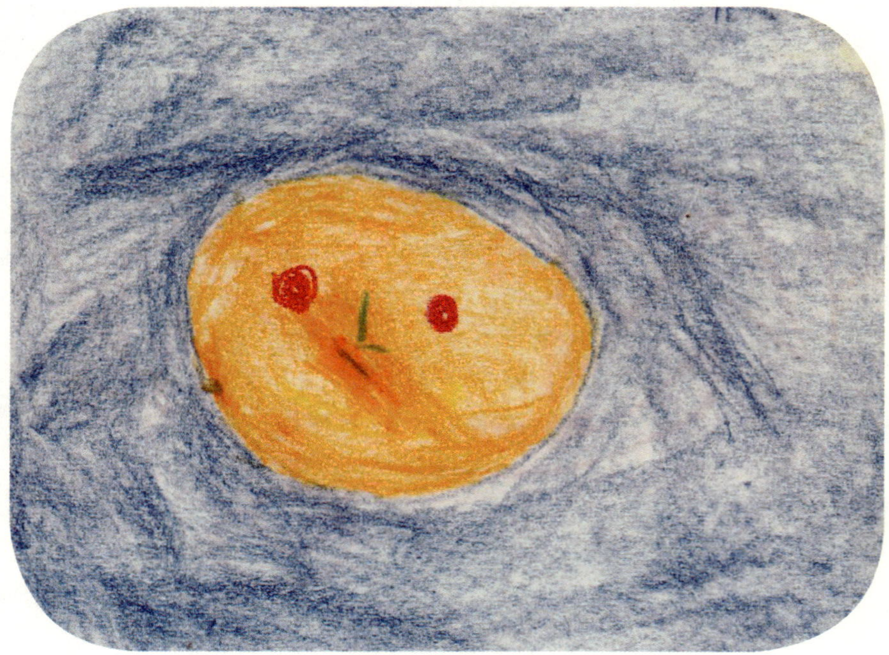

The Tabula Smaragdina

Over a period of many years, I frequently was confronted with the hermetic knowledge contained in the Tabula Smaragdina. This work is written as a postulate of twelve short statements. The turgid writing of Hermes Trismegistus was repeatedly put aside until the Child Artist introduced the illustration of the Three Kings. Was this a subconscious intent? The connection of the symbolic picture with the old wisdom of Egypt becomes the bridge spanning at least three thousand years.

Nevertheless, our Child Artist could not possibly have knowledge of Hermes Trismegistus except through memories from his past lives. Because I feel that the source of his proclivity is derived from the resources with which he was born, I listened to his introduction and heeded his information that would become the scaffold of this book. It is the Child Artist who leads us to examine alchemy and embryology, or embryogenesis. The content of the postulate II to XI of the Emerald Tablet will be examined to explain the writings and sketches throughout this book.

We introduce the great mythical figure known as *Thoth,* the deity whose wisdom exceeded all other Gods, Pharaohs, and Priests ruling over that region. He adopted the earthly name Hermes Trismegistus, which appears in the history of the Sumerian people, Hellenistic culture, and Egyptian tombs as a hieroglyph. This earthly dweller introduces himself as "The Three in One," the thrice anointed, the knower of the past, present, and future, initiated with the knowledge of the Heavens, the Earth, and the human being. He was exalted by his students as a being of great wisdom and a master of healing. He became known throughout the ages as the greatest philosopher, priest, and king.

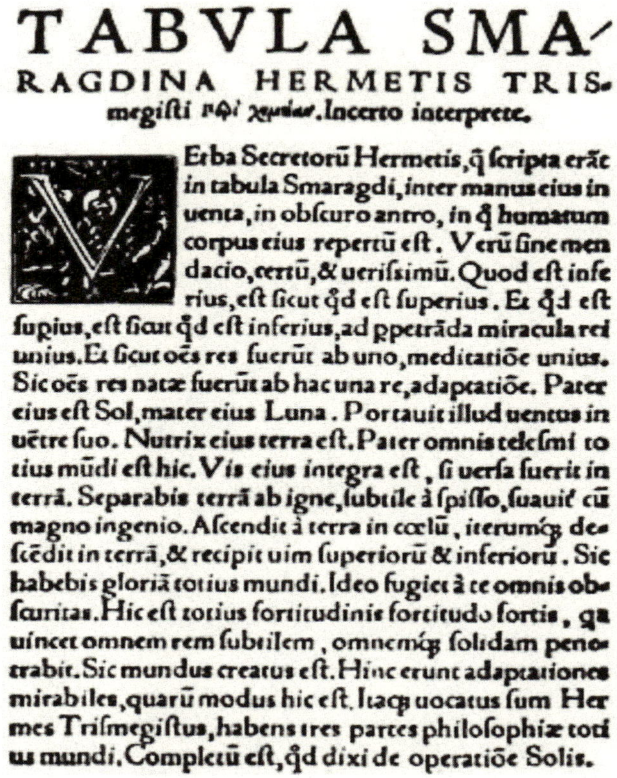

TABVLA SMA-
RAGDINA HERMETIS TRIS-
megiſti περὶ χημείας. Incerto interprete.

VErba Secretorū Hermetis, q̄ ſcripta erāt
in tabula Smaragdi, inter manus eius in
uenta, in obſcuro antro, in q̄ humatum
corpus eius repertū eſt. Verū ſine men
dacio, certū, & ueriſsimū. Quod eſt infe
rius, eſt ſicut q̄d eſt ſuperius. Et q̄d eſt
ſupius, eſt ſicut q̄d eſt inferius, ad ppetrāda miracula rei
unius. Et ſicut oēs res fuerūt ab uno, meditatiōe unius.
Sic oēs res natæ fuerūt ab hac una re, adaptatiōe. Pater
eius eſt Sol, mater eius Luna. Portauit illud uentus in
uētre ſuo. Nutrix eius terra eſt. Pater omnis teleſmi to
tius mūdi eſt hic. Vis eius integra eſt, ſi uerſa fuerit in
terrā. Separabis terrā ab igne, ſubtile à ſpiſſo, ſuauit' cū
magno ingenio. Aſcendit à terra in cœlū, iterumq; de-
ſcēdit in terrā, & recipit uim ſuperiorū & inferiorū. Sic
habebis gloriā totius mundi. Ideo fugiet à te omnis ob-
ſcuritas. Hic eſt totius fortitudinis fortitudo fortis, quia
uincet omnem rem ſubtilem, omnemq; ſolidam pene-
trabit. Sic mundus creatus eſt. Hinc erunt adaptationes
mirabiles, quarū modus hic eſt. Itaq; uocatus ſum Her
mes Triſmegiſtus, habens tres partes philoſophiæ toti
us mundi. Completū eſt, q̄d dixi de operatiōe Solis.

Plate 25: Tabula smaragdina (Latin text)

Hermes Trismegistus is purported to have written numerous tracts, the best known of which is called *Tabulae Smaragdina,* or Emerald Tablet. It contains twelve cryptic postulates, which were translated in Latin and widely quoted and studied by students of

THE TABULA SMARAGDINA (English)

I True, True. Without doubt. Certain.

II The below is as the above, and the above as the below, to perfect the wonders of **The One**.

III And as all things came from *the One*, from the meditation of *the One*, so, too, all things are born from this *One* by adaptation.

IV Its father is the Sun; its mother is the Moon; the Wind carries it in its belly; its nurse is the Earth.

V It is the father of all the wonders of the whole world. Its power is perfect when it is transformed into earth.

VI Separate the earth from fire and the subtle from the gross, cautiously and judiciously.

VII It ascends from the Earth to Heaven, and then returns back to the Earth, so that it receives the power of the upper and the lower.

VIII Thus you will possess the brightness of the whole world, and all darkness will flee you.

IX This is the force of all forces, for it overcomes all that is subtle, and penetrates solid things.

X Thus the world was created.

XI From this, wonderful adaptations are effected, and the means are given here.

XII And Hermes Trismegistus is my name, because I possess the three parts of the wisdom of the whole world.

alchemy throughout the past 1,500 years. Even in English, the true meaning behind this writing was not clear to me when I studied it twenty years ago. Subjectively, I found the statements presented in the tablet somewhat bombastic and obtuse and the development of the postulates difficult to grasp.

Thanks to my thorough study that followed my examination of the drawing "Initiation of the Three Kings," I have revised my callous judgment of years ago. Here we will introduce the statements of that document as it was handed down from antiquity. The whole document appears earlier for readers to study. It was only through the Child Artist introduction of the Three Kings picture that I took a renewed interest in the hermetic or alchemical knowledge humanity has been working on for three thousand years without much success in clarifying the text satisfactorily. After being reintroduced to this text through the Child Artist and his Three Kings drawings, I reached another conclusion.

It is easy for modern minds to reject most ancient writings, to judge older texts subjectively, in an attitude of arrogance and cynicism. These initiated human beings, wise with the information of the vertical, spiritual plane, were able to convey spiritual knowledge to religious centers of the world starting with Tibet, India, Persia, and Sumerian civilization. However they were still under a mandate of secrecy and were adept at writing symbolic texts. With the closing of the Iron Age esoteric material is becoming increasingly available for all to read, including on Wikipedia.

Quality of Numbers

One—the Sophia

Medjugorje, June 24, 1981: An apparition occurred in Bosnia, close to the Croatian border and 108 miles northeast of the Adriatic Sea. Six teenagers in the small town of Medjugorje were introduced to a feminine presence, which I will call an "unidentified atmospheric phenomenon" (plate 23). Although all the participants in this chosen group experienced unsettling fear and emotional instability, their visits to a stony outcrop named Mount Podbrdo continued for a few weeks after the summer solstice at a certain time each day, a few hours before sunset. All of the visionaries had a Catholic upbringing, and it was purported that messages were exchanged. According to the local population, the visions involved the Madonna. Worldwide interest was stimulated by occurrences of spontaneous healing and testimonials of objects being transformed into gold. Beginning in 1986, trips from North America were organized. The region of Bosnia and Herzegovina was ruled by a communist regime at the time, and the phenomenon was unpopular with the local government, which did everything it could to halt the influx of tourists. Many photos of the phenomenon can be found on the Internet. The picture included here was given to me by a visitor to the sight in 1986. At that time Kodak films were still used. It was the owner of the camera who received the gift of "the sight." Her sharing made it possible to publicly announce the new reality of these etheric phenomena and the visage's true identity as the Gaia/Maya, and the "Soul of Human." On examination of this picture my subjective first impression was one of awe and heart silence. How pure this being, how exquisite in her beauty, her mature youthfulness, and her feminine wholeness. Could the eye of the artist ever imitate such a representation on canvas? If so I never had seen a painting even come close to such an uplifting image, an image that fortified my knowing and full acceptance of the previously described phenomenon.

Plate 26: Sophia photographic imprint

What came through on the sensitive photographic film is the "etheric" print of a feminine figure. It is not a solid representation of a woman. The backdrop, seen through the figure, is the mountain as seen from the hotel window. Even the parking lot or a road on the hotel grounds can be identified through the hem of the dress. Of all the pictures taken by visitors to the site, this image is unique and can be seen on many websites.

The visionaries identify this apparition as a holy member of the Catholic hierarchy, which becomes a subjective issue. *"She"* does not exist for the Holy See alone but is there for all of humanity, because She is an aspect connected to the human soul. In our description of the Gnostic myth, we identify her as Gaya.

In any case, the phenomena of "etheric visions" need to be recognized as objective fact. More human beings throughout the world have experienced "sights," and in this instance she was identified as the eternal feminine presence who accompanies humanity in its evolution.

Throughout centuries the Madonna has been adored when intercession in personal life was fervently requested. Visions of the LADY have been recorded throughout the world. A major proponent for these phenomena are the members of the Roman Church directed by the Holy See. Naming her, the Madonna is a natural response, but not correct. The visions are seen in the atmosphere and are phenomenologically correct. The content of the atmosphere varies under changing conditions. The reflection is seen in air having high humidity. Reflective qualities of atmospheric metals like silver and gold are carried and make this etheric phenomenon possible. Soon atmospheric visions will not be proclaimed only by the "religious" section of humanity. These unidentified atmospheric phenomena will become objectively scientifically proven, at that moment Natural Science will embrace the etheric organization of the living world. The proof will be searched for through the pressure of the ordinary person and scientists themselves, who become witnesses and demand a qualitative expansion of the world. More and more people will speak out of knowing, which is also *witnessing,* not belief.

Twofold

An article by Katalin Balog in *The New York Times,* "'Son of Saul,' Kierkegaard, and the Holocaust" (Feb. 28, 2016), elegantly introduces the concept that the Danish philosopher Søren Kierkegaard (1813–1855) called *existentialism.* The film *Son of Saul* prompted her to make an intimate assessment of the emotional crisis faced by modern human beings. Kierkegaard observed the growing tendency toward an objective abstract perspective of the world, opposing considerations of the spiritual richness and lawful heritage of each human being. These two radical, opposing worldviews were thoroughly delineated by existentialism. The dual capacity of the human being to interpret the world as abstraction (purely from a horizontal orientation), while taking into account the inner experience of the conscious life, is threatened by existentialism, which emerged after World War II with the writings of Jean Paul Sartre, who stated that each of us exists as an individual in a purposeless universe, and that we must oppose our hostile environment by exercising our free will. Objectivity or subjectivity—both human experiences—were evaluated by natural scientists with the result that

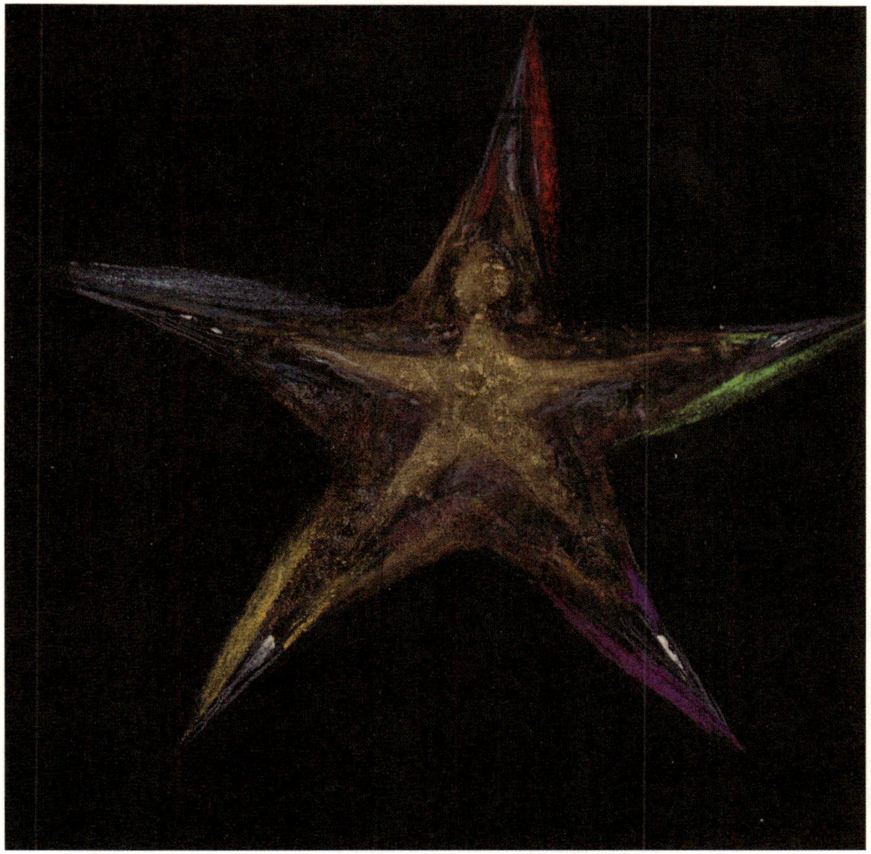

Plate 27: Infinite heritage

subjectivity, intuition, inner conviction, and imaginations—all the rich inner feelings—became unacceptable in the presentation of scientific papers.

To Rudolf Steiner, the imbalanced soul development with which humanity was threatened could be compensated by the recognition that a child enters world existence not with a blank slate (*tabula rasa*), but as a product of reincarnation and therefore of considerable value to the evolution of humanity. Steiner called the extensive body of knowledge that he shared through books, lectures, and drawings "Anthroposophy," or wisdom of the human being. Anthroposophy is a spiritual science and shares a place with the Eastern religious philosophies—Theosophy, Buddhism, Hinduism, and so on. The mystery of the life and death of the Christ is at the core of many of his lectures. Rosicrucianism and esoteric Christianity were inaugurated at the beginning of the twentieth century.

Exercising living thinking becomes a tool in comprehending the concepts in Spiritual Science. The aspiring student must become familiar with the two orientations toward the world. Naming and experiencing polarities, for instance, is the first step toward an imagination in evaluating two worlds. As a routine exercise, one begins by creating two columns, each headed by a noun or adjective for which an opposite condition exists.

The beauty of this exercise is the possibility it affords us to find a position between these two realities that reflects a place to identify one's self. The horizontal reality is the world in which we live, a reality that is finite and conditioned to our existence on Earth. On Earth, I identify myself as a person with a name, address, position, status, and so on. On the vertical plane I exist but as an individual hardly known to myself. Even my gender has no impact on my vertical existence. One has to question whether the unknown vertical dimension can be explored through the study of Spiritual Science and how it can be done.

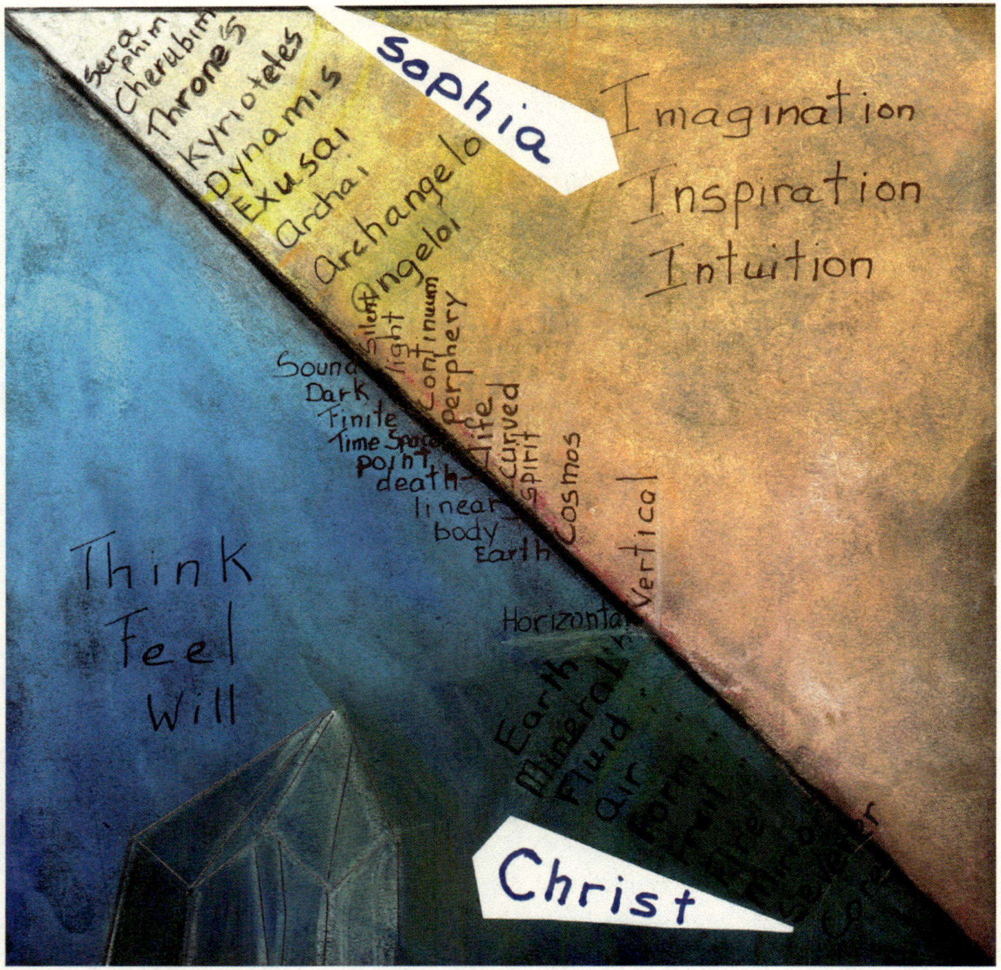

Plate 28: Horizontal versus vertical planes of reality

As we move into the third millennium, much pertains to functions exercised on what I like to call the horizontal plane—knowledge accumulated through use of the five senses, one's memories, and the soul capacities of thinking, feeling, and will activity. On this plane, ever more information is gathered. Memory does not have to be activated; all is obtainable through the Internet. A scientist triumphs through knowledge accumulated during the short time on Earth. Matter, distances, calculations, molecular reactions in the laboratory and so on, pertain to the life in vitro and to existences beyond our universe. Today we even have knowledge of the constitution of genes, viruses, and prions. We have yet to penetrate the secret of life (*in vivo*) and to create life out of nothingness as only the gods can do. We remain limited to the horizontal plane, limited in time and limited in our awareness of the vertical plane.

The vertical plane as a different dimension has remained hidden until only a century ago, when the wisdom of these existences were revealed to random members of humanity who were sensitive to auditory and visual stimuli streaming in from the vertical plane. Eastern and Western masters of religious practices have been able to teach their followers about the vertical dimensions throughout the ages, but such knowledge requires rigorous physical and mental practices. Freedom is in the differences between spontaneous information flowing toward me from another dimension and the information I gain from a master. That inner voice I hear still leaves me with a choice of action or non-action. By submitting to the direction of a meditative practice I feel less free but more triumphant with results and information that may be manipulated.

The intricacies of the vertical plane are difficult to grasp for those who remain unaware or skeptical of its existence. The more I learn on the physical plane, the more my capacities for imaginations are blunted. Listening to "others" requires a capacity of silencing my own voice of judgment, objection, and disagreement. Just Listen! Imagine This! Conceiving this plane as an infinite entity, I experience myself as an eternal being. Time has no beginning, no end. Space is not empty, on the contrary, having silenced my own head-chatter, information flows in and through me; cosmic thoughts think in me. It's as if I become the instrument for or in the vertical plane. I think speech; I speak; I have spoken. The gods have spoken. It would be frivolous to think that it is *"I"* or *my* thought manifest. On this vertical plane, I become the instrument for the gods' messengers, entities belonging to the as-yet unknown hierarchies from stars, universes, and other dimensions beyond.

I see humanity tapping into knowledge of the vertical plane and wisdom of infinite space, the progression from warmth to life, our role in evolution of humanity as bearers of love and freedom, and the final amalgamation of all humanity to become light bearers.

Placing the two planes at right angles to each other and experiencing my place on each of these planes is a good exercise. The future makes ascent on the vertical arrow between the two planes an enticing possibility. With a controlled soul life achieving balance in the functions of thought, feeling, and will, one gains the ability to place oneself on a higher rung of the ladder while participating fully on the horizontal plane.

The secrets of "the tree of knowledge" will be revealed to humanity in times to come, as may be seen in the younger generations, who reveal this knowing in a symbolic language. My personal experience of meeting these revelations has become a part of this book.

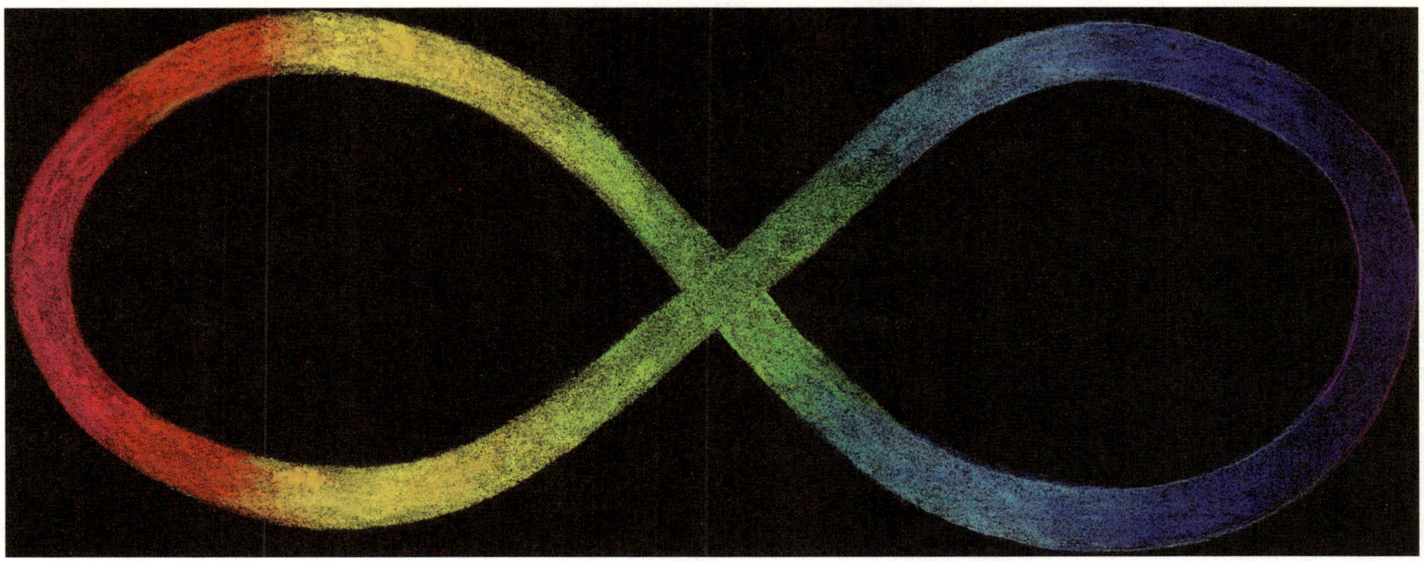

Plate 29: Equilibrium of two poles establishes health

Threefold

The progression of values from two to three includes the awareness that a center exists between two polarities. Here we can insert the symbol of infinity that is able to express a pendulum motion, beautifully expressed in our colorful drawing (plate 29).

A rhythm is established with movement between poles. Rhythm is life. Stepping into the living world one immediately recognizes the presence of a threefold order, polar opposites, and the balance in between. In the plant world we project these three distinct divisions such as root system for absorption of nutrients, the leaves for the respiration and circulation in the plant, and finally the flower and seed formation as a method for reproduction. There is an obvious correlation between this scaffolding of the plant and the human body. The Child Artist when asked to draw a person draws himself as a flower rooted in the earth (see plate 3). In the following table we can demonstrate that this threefolding finds a parallel in the characteristics of the three regions so that we can identify ourselves as an upside-down plant.

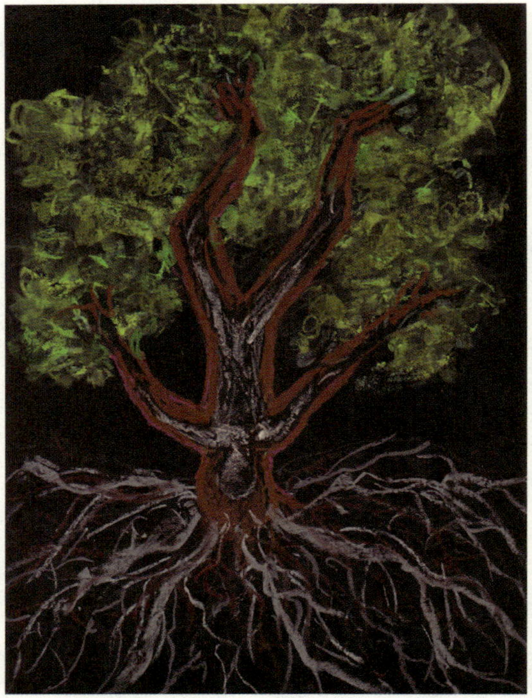

Plate 30: Plant as upside down human

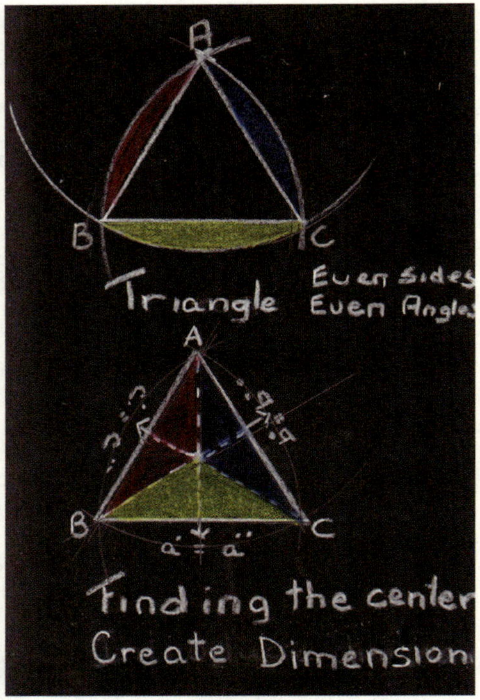

Plate 31: Triangle and additional dimension

Threefold Order as Reflected in Human-beings

Root	Protection in earth	Stationary	Uptake of salt crystals	Nervous system
Leaf	Exposure to atmosphere	Rhythmic	Gas exchange	Pulmonary / Respiratory system(s)
Flower	Invaded by visitors	Chaotic	Excretion of substance	Muscular / Digestion / Reproductive system(s)

As early as the education in Greek temples, students were introduced to the triangle and the laws that were established out of the subject of trigonometry. The triangle was envisioned as a flat dimension. However when a fourth dimension was contemplated, the student moved into the concept of four folding adding the next step to the conception of space, depth, and the reality of progression to more intricate space occupying figures (Pythagorean solids).

The spiritual counterpart was also significant for the young students with the recognition that a parallel existed in the vertical world, the world of deities from the stars, where knowledge of the human being presented itself with a unique spirit, personified with character and manifesting in a physical body. Spirit-soul-body, a division of three; that is what was learned.

Fourfold

Standing on Earth, the personal experience of the body is on four planes—the front, the back, the left, and the right. All living creatures starting with the plant kingdom do have a relationship with the four elements that belong to the earth, mineral, water, air, and fire. The culmination of the evolutionary process on Earth is the human species also called Homo Erectus. We are the fourth Kingdom. This placement is attained through the capacity to reason while combining the soul-instruments of thought, emotions, and a will to act. While in the process of reasoning, human beings organize their environment, which enables them to bring order. In the evolutionary process, progression from sentience to intellectual exploration followed by an awakened consciousness is witnessed.

The cadaver consists of the minerals found in the elementary table. Since the days of Aristotle (383–323 BC) Western culture recognizes four elements that constitute the living world. They are called earth (solid minerals); water (fluids); air and light; and fire and warmth. In Asian cultures, wood is another constituent named as an element. The four intertwined principles present themselves in the animal and human kingdoms. Constantly ordering the living world through the functions of this division lends order in the domain of functions.

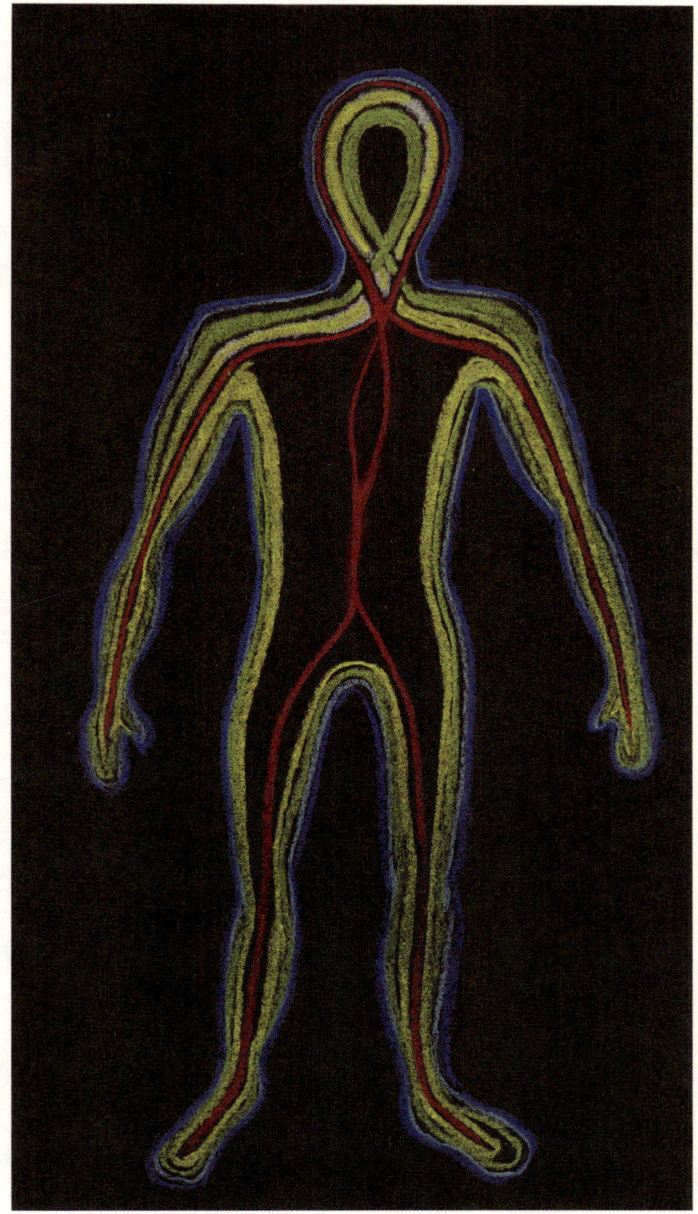

Plate 32: Fourfold permeating body

Hierarchies of Earth

Kingdom	Examples
Human	Homo Erectus
Animal	Evolution from water to land Insects Bacteria
Plant	Evolution from one cell
Mineral	Virus Atoms providing solidity

Through Spiritual Science, we learn that the physical body in its living presentation is suffused with three subtler bodies. We could also imagine that the solid mineral earth body is penetrated by a water body, an air body that carries light, and a warmth body. This is indeed so, come to think about it, otherwise the volume of ninety percent water weight would make us unable to move with such alacrity, ease, and ebullience. The body of water is a living entity and contains within it again the fourfold expression of life-warmth, light, tone, and life. Naming these bodies has a specific purpose insofar as the name connects these subtler bodies with our surroundings. The etheric body refers to life itself, with the water as a stepping-stone; no water, no life. The astral body would then refer to the stars we identify at night, so that what the cosmic extension presents with its planets and stars imbues us, becoming part and parcel of the emotional psyche, conscious or unconscious.

In addition to life, the animal kingdom must experience movement and emotion to survive adverse stimuli from the environment. Whereas animals can guard themselves from cold or heat, human beings have to develop a skill for regulating their own heat exchange, including skills in making clothing and housing. Over thousands of years, the "I" has evolved so that the once-dominant sentient quality has been replaced by intellect and consciousness. Evolution from earthliness to saintliness is vouchsafed.

The Earth itself is divided in four kingdoms—mineral, plant, animal, and human kingdoms all have places in the destiny, and hence the evolution, of this planet. Past, present, and future are interwoven in these four representations of the kingdoms, or hierarchies. Humanity cannot separate itself from the other kingdoms, since we are interdependent. Human beings are seen as the culmination in the evolution of life on this planet, but the accomplishment of its ultimate goal still lies far into the future.

Fivefold

These five vowels (*A E I O U*) have an evolutionary quality. Using these qualities in the sequence of the sections with which we introduce the story of creation as a mythical, subjective experience will help explain the Child Artist's sketches.

Observe how speech in young children is an art that needs to be acquired. When around a baby, adults are always willing to imitate and demonstrate the infant's first words, and we may notice that the words are rich with "ah" vowels in all languages. I have a strong image of how the human larynx differs from the ape-man prototype in its width of the hyoid bone. Not only did the skull extend in size, but the larynx was also prepared as the organ for speech. The first incarnations of human souls had to mold the laryngeal structure and the mandible so that the tool for speech could develop. My imaginative picture shows the air filled in the evening with women's voices around the fires, toning the vowels as in a song and freeing the air trapped in their bodies. The children who were not asleep joined the choir in a communal gesture of gratitude. The first recorded stories appear eons later, when humanity had evolved to form communities, a multitude of languages, the art of writing and scientific explorations. All these endeavors were guided by the centers of religion, in which priests controlled information and steered the population into servitude. Members of the royalty were seen as god-humans and were deified, unreachable, and the ultimate leaders of priests and humanity.

All sounds of the earth, water, and atmosphere carry outward (centrifugal) from the source through vibrations and pulsing percussion. When no substance exists, as in a vacuum, vibrations cannot be carried. Water is the best conductor of sound vibrations. The vast volume of the seas is made smaller by excellent sound conduction, allowing sea mammals to remain in contact with one another over great distances and depths.

The ear as a sense organ accomplishes hearing. It is equipped to capture incoming vibrations through air as well as more deeply within the skull through lymphatic fluid. The quality of vibrations we hear is twofold. First, we can hear tone created by a musical instrument or singing birds; the vibrations travel through air. In addition, speech and sound have different qualities. The vibrations created by the organs for speech (the larynx, the mouth, and nasal spaces) are evaluated continuously by the one who recreates the words, hearing the vowels and consonants through the conduction of fluid spaces around the pharynx and inner ear. It is fascinating that the words I form with the speech organ have a dual purpose. Spoken words travel through the waters in my own body and affect the formative forces, also called the tone or chemical ethers of the "etheric" body. The influence on the finer, astral and etheric bodies, including the emotions, are decisive. Vowels and consonants representing the concept *The Word* are imbued with creative force. Furthermore, speech becomes an instrument for contact

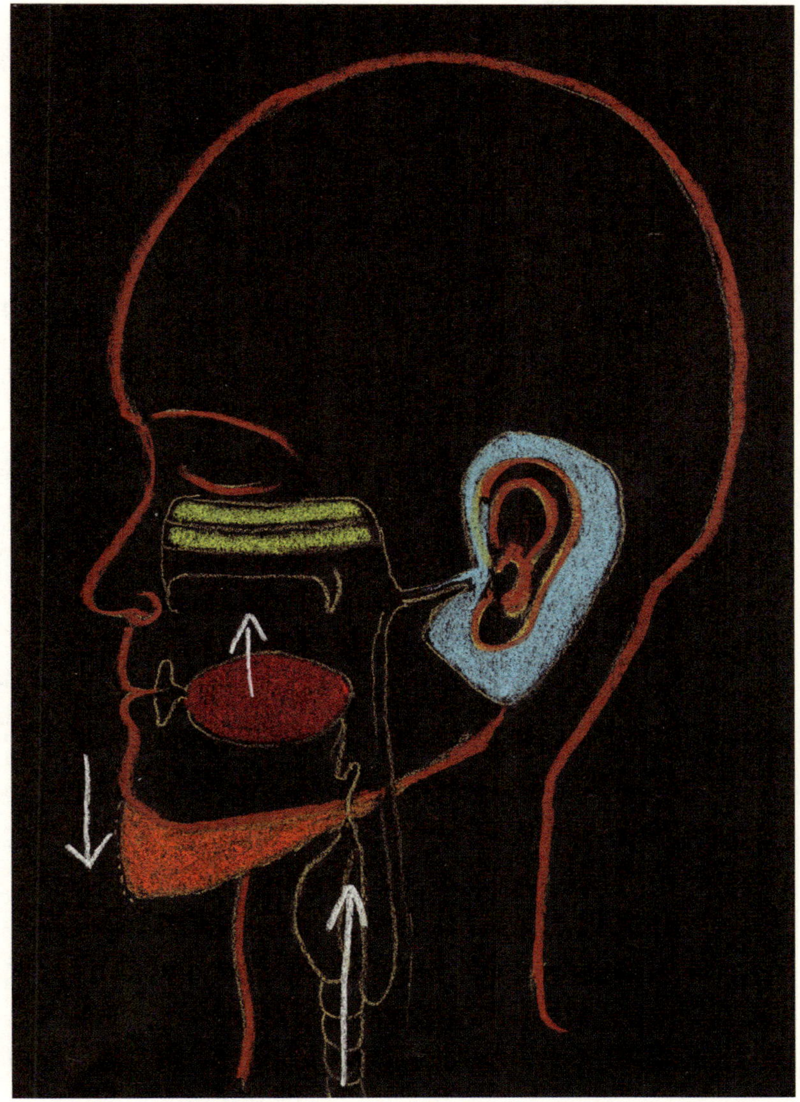

Plate 33: Space for vowel sounds

with other human beings and, throughout the evolution, has been a powerful instrument for building communities and cultures.

All of humanity has a relationship to vowels. Although each language writes the pure sound differently, the act of forming them remains the same. When forming a pure *A* ("ah"), the mouth opens wide, the mandible drops with the tongue pressed against the lower jaw, and the cheeks are drawn sideways. This is the sound doctors request to examine the throat. With the *E* sound ("ey"), the jaw is pulled up slightly as the tongue makes a platform for the sound to role off. This sound is often used in a staccato and provides a defensive barrier. The next sound, *I* ("ee"), can be formed by squeezing the jaw and mouth space tightly with the tongue. The *O* ("oh") sound is produced by a hollow space with jaw, tongue, even the palate. The *U* ("oo") formation requires tightening the facial muscles, tongue, and jaw. The ultimate holy vowel is the combination of *A* and *U,* finishing with *M*. This sequence of vowel and consonant is practiced by the monks in chorus and fosters a meditative mood of reverence and a true conversation with the heavens.

As suggested, the vowels work on the human physical organism, which consists of minerals (9%) and liquids (91%). The effect of each vowel is specific, and with careful observation human beings experience a specific vibrational flow in the organism. We have to imagine that the column of water representing my human body is inundated with the sounding of an particular vowel sound, and in consciousness my "I" responds to that experience. With *Ah* sounding, the human body (column of living water) opens up to what surrounds it. What is outside is allowed to enter, expand, and fill me. Its gesture inspires me; it becomes a deep experience of adoration and desire to be one with all.

In the sound expression of *E* ("ey"), a flowing motion is established as an exhalation occurs. I exist as a polarity of right and left and crossing of the two opposites. Through this, I establish boundaries expressed in the warning of the staccato sound "hey." This sound is twofold: streaming and interruption. The point of interruption, or silence, creates room for a new condition. This is a creative sound.

The next vowel, *I* as expressed in sound ("ee"), has a definitive upright radiating gesture. The gestalt *I* experience is the presence of light flowing from the earth on which I stand. It fortifies my inner being and is expressed by limbs outstretched with inner light toward my surroundings. I raise my lower jaw; my sounding wants to be heard. I AM. I am infinite. I incarnate. I am immortal. I am an individuality.

In the *O* ("oh"), my organism resounds toward an enfolding embrace of the outside world; I incorporate the other. The other and I are ONE. I am not alone. I as a person can hold hands with another person.

The last vowel, the *U* ("oo") sound, is distinct from the other sounds and imbues a specific experience. It is an astringent posturing extension of uprightness. It holds itself contained in my gestalt so that I can reach beyond the stars with my acumen. It actually enables me to extend myself into the cosmic infinity. It is a sound for the future, Utopia, the universe, the commune of searchers, and the sound of Spirit.

Sixfold: Contribution of Speech

The human being through its speech acquires creative powers. This will manifest as a conscious asset in the future. The six positions of the body and limbs in space convey the connection to the spoken word and its importance to **The One**.

In the first sequence, plate 34, the time element for the "I" is introduced. Here the "I" experiences itself on the horizontal plane.

In the final three postures, plate 35, reaching for the vertical plane in space completes the potential of **The One.**

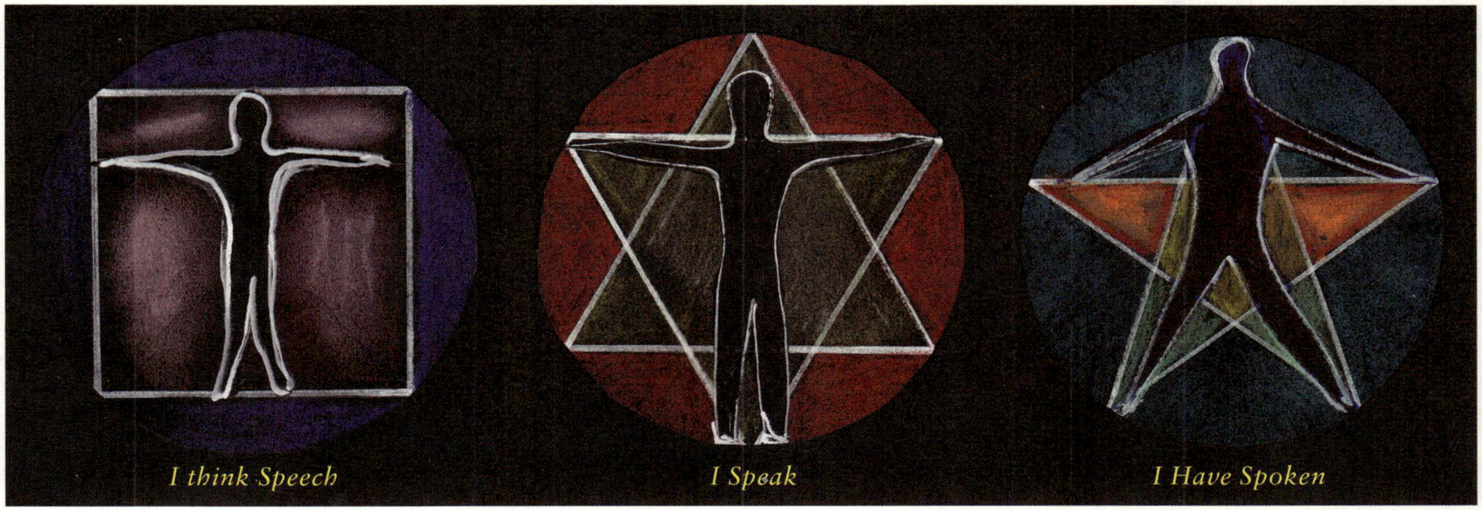
I think Speech
I Speak
I Have Spoken

Plate 34: Horizontal time element of speech

Past Creating through the Word

Present Creating through Goodness

Future Creating through Love

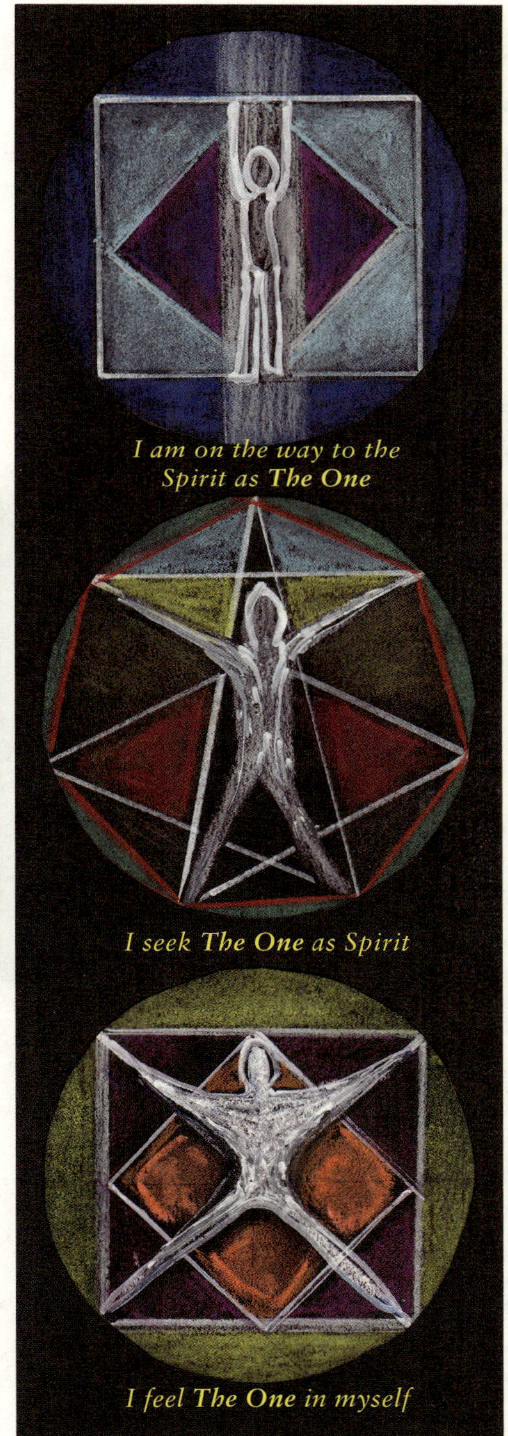
I am on the way to the Spirit as The One
I seek The One as Spirit
I feel The One in myself

Plate 35:Vertical space element of speech

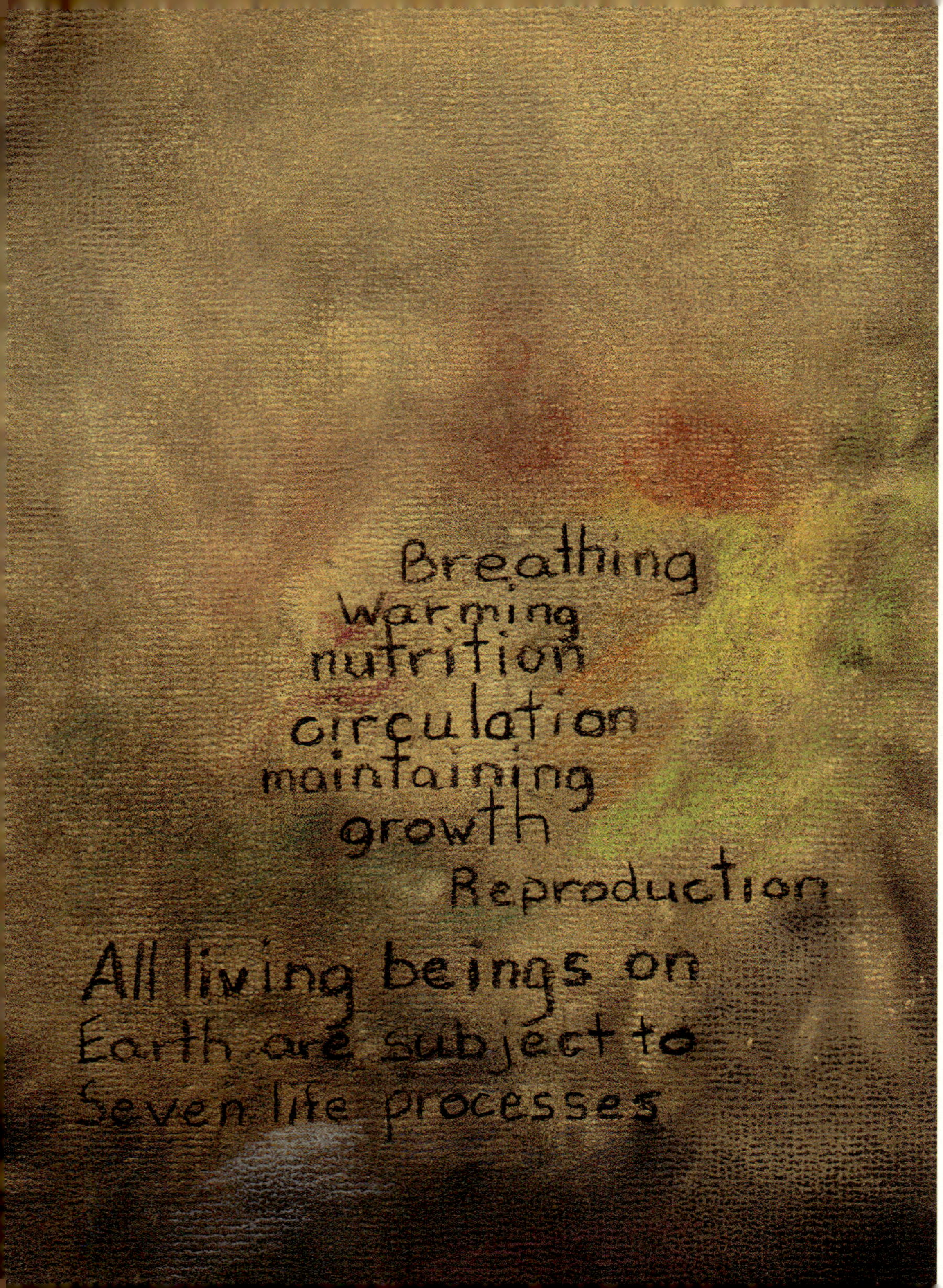

Sevenfold—Life on Earth

Seven life processes are embedded in the specie evolution as observed on Earth. Our dynamic earthly lives bear witness to this haunting fact. To envision polarities of life and death and the phases in between these realities of nature, brings home the ineffability of an environment where life is not possible. Life is present starting from the human kingdom down to the plant kingdom. On Earth all living cell structures are subject to seven life processes.

In the evolution of life forms we do not see a slow accumulation or acquisition of these processes over millions of years. They are present from the start. Even in the single-cell amoeba, all seven life processes penetrate the existence of beginnings.

These processes are: breathing, warming, nutrition, circulation, maintaining, growth, and reproduction. One can reason that the template for life exists from the beginning. Form and function will evolve to adjust to the environment, but the integrity of the processes is steadfast and no functions are lost.

Was this template brought to the Earth?

Could the introduction of the template be performed by the human being for the human being who after all is the highest evolutionary being on Earth?

Plate 36: The seven life processes

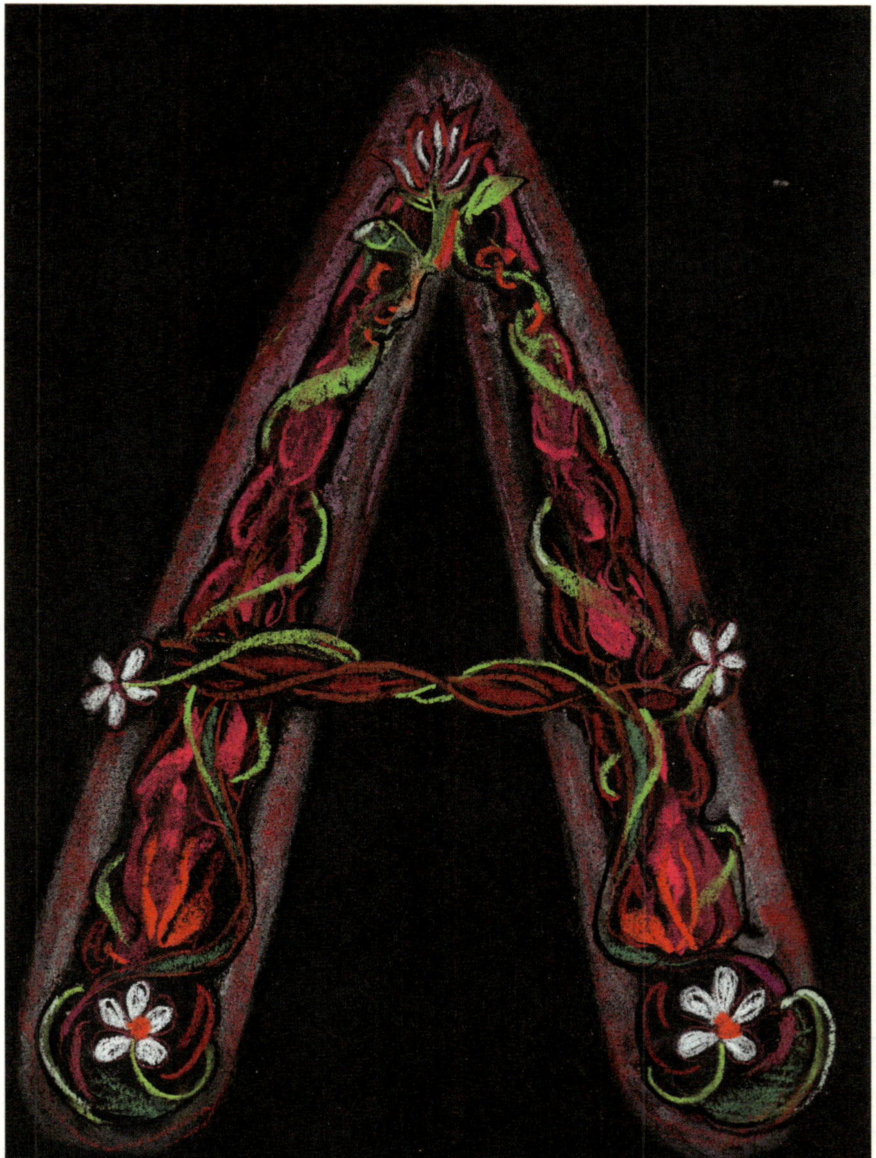

Plate 37: Sound A as depiction

Sound A

The first section appearing under the energy of the "ah" vowel is dedicated to the first knowledge given to and accumulated by ancient humanity—knowledge of nature phenomena, the secrets of plants and their use in healing, and the domestication of animals to enrich the food chain.

An abundance of images come to consciousness in the expression of this vowel. *Ah,* as sung by a choir of pure voices, is a celestial sound that grounds human beings with a wide stance on the Earth, steadfastly, but able to reach out into the immediate surroundings with slowly raising arms in a gesture of embrace and exultation. Abundance of life, joy of experiencing the Sun's light, warmth found in the company of other beings around night fires—all could contribute to repetitive imitation of this sound through modulation of the vocal chords. This took place in temples as religious centers, where the population found leadership, protection, and guidance for millennia.

Among the youth, children with exceptional qualities were invited to join the temple schooling with a promise of future leadership. Temple science was dedicated to the introduction of pupils to the quality of substances, discussions on evaluating subjective soul experiences during their rigorous studies, and guiding pupils in demonstrating their understanding through artistic representations. The disciplines to which pupils of both genders were familiarized included the secrets of life and death through manipulating nature, obedience to a recognized hierarchy, and the cultivation of nobility. The goal of education concerned the development of feelings of wonder connected to deities, nature spirits, and the discarnate soul of their master. Self-development

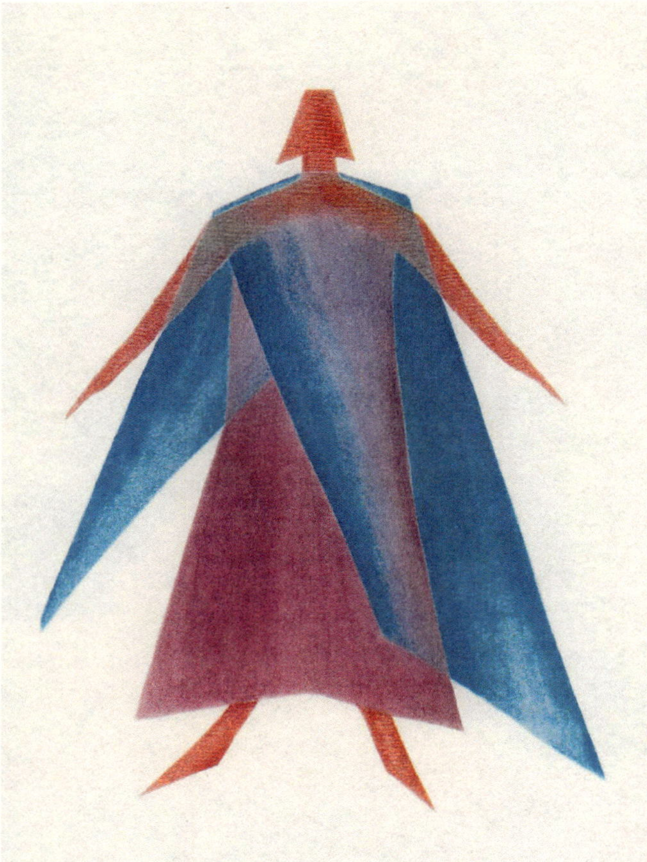

Plate 38: Eurythmy gesture of A

was encouraged, so that a future responsibility, empathy for life, and emotional restraint became second nature for the future earthly leaders. Many branches of discipline were embraced.

Throughout the ages, the content of these treasured lessons metamorphosed. What once was then accepted with the highest esteem has now become scorned science—*alchemy,* thoroughly replaced by modern quantitative sciences dedicated solely to the physical reality of a horizontal world. Pupils on their path of exploration researched the beingness *"qual"* of substance, connecting first of all with the polarities in nature—the processes of decay and death versus the abundance of life and growth.

Primitive human beings could choose between two worlds. The still-dormant sentient soul life of human beings was guided by "teachers" in centers placed at strategic points throughout evolving and expanding human population. In contrast to members of the animal kingdom, the human constitution was such that there was an inherent quest to dominate the outer world. It reminds one of the paradisaical tale—humanity at a crossing between stagnancy or expansion and exploration.

There were two realities: The rich, protected, inner world of self-realization or the ambitious daring and stimulating path of discovering new worlds—"where no man has gone before." Human soul potential manifested in the polarities of love and hate and the corresponding responses of attraction or rejection. The existence of contrast became the leading evolutionary impetus leading humankind to prefer and choose the "horizontal" world dimensions of illusionary material possession, the desire to feel superior, and the will to oppress and dominate.

In the older civilizations such as India, we can still find remnants of people with opposite persuasions—the holy men and women and ascetics who lead lives dedicated to self-exploration, inner equilibrium, and dedication to the objective reality of higher dimensions beyond the horizontal plane.

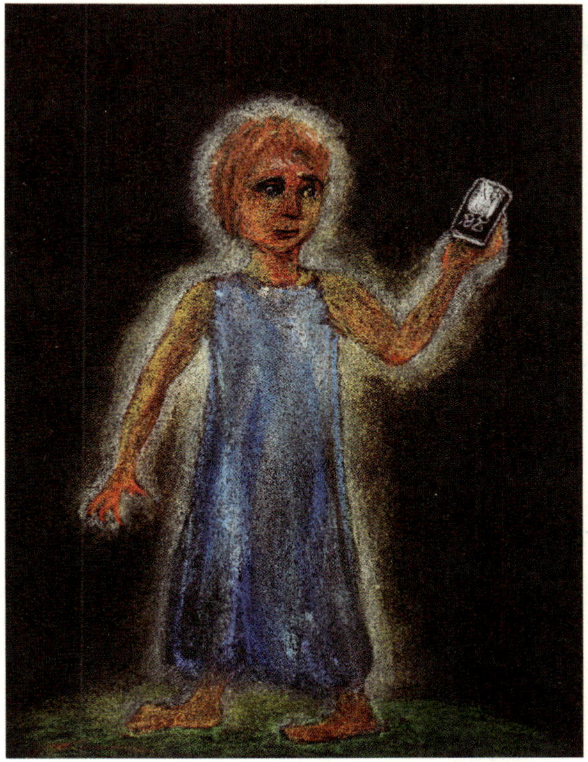

Plate 39: Distraction

For those schooled in ancient monasteries, dedication to poverty, chastity, and obedience became the standard for schooling in control of the soul functions of thinking, feeling, and the will. Surrounded by a chaotic world of cacophony and fear, human beings increasingly search for an inner journey that promises silence and bliss together with the knowledge of higher worlds. Aspirations to attain knowledge or become conscious of an alternate "vertical" plane, indicates a swing of the pendulum.

Poverty	Modest humble in self	Thinking
Chastity	Containment of emotions	Feeling
Obedience	Following the greater good	Will

The introduction of electronic screens into modern civilization within the last fifty years of human evolution is remarkable. Those of the post-World War II generation have all been captivated by screen images alien to reality. The temptation of advertising and absurd entertainment is welcomed distraction to daily social and family interactions. As long as these images dominate the consciousness of the children, their own human potential remains unexplored. In the last ten years, teachers have to compete with personal screens brought to school by children who prefer to communicate with one another through texting. Satisfaction with the entertainment and even an addiction to the illusionary distraction will become a primary source of frustration in educational goals for humanity. The use of personal screens and audio devices captivates the human senses, which become seduced by images of intense, nonexistent virtual reality. The potential danger of using electromagnetic media hour after hour by all of humanity cannot be ignored. For most people, possessing and using screens during their waking hours of the day becomes a distraction and, consequently, a negation and denial of their own powers of exploring the human mind and the development of inner capacities.

The powers of imagination are an inherent human capacity great potential. Training the imagination of a developing young human being is the greatest responsibility in the educational curriculum. It is clear that students trained in imagination will also acquire tools for inspiration and intuition, created from their own inner experience. Children learning to focus on one impression at a time, whether an image, a song, or a musical instrument, will be stimulated to identify truth, beauty, and goodness through the recognition that such human potential indeed exists. Training imagination by focusing the five senses in creating living pictures is essential for awaking and strengthening the capacities

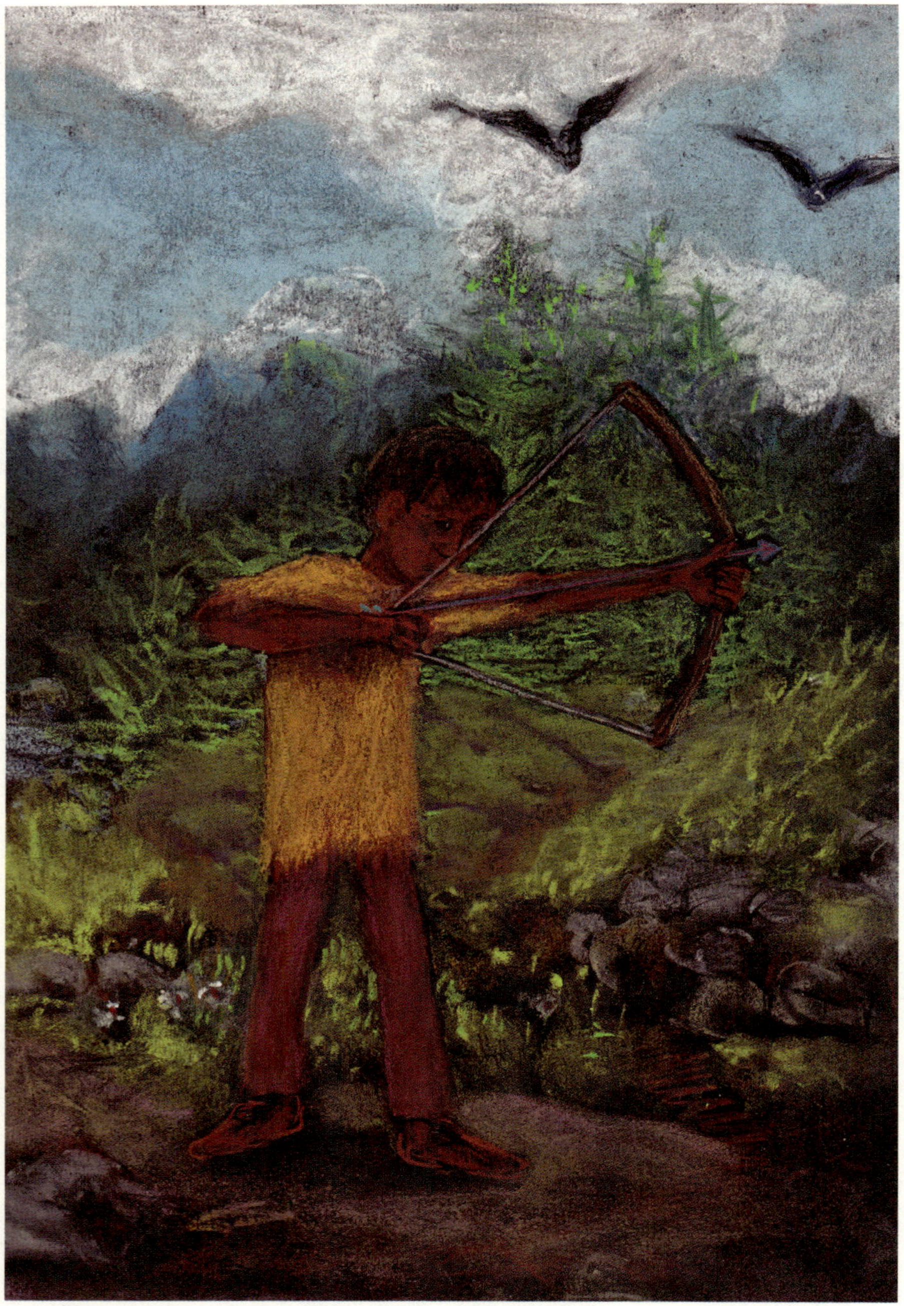

of children to explore these truths. Knowledge gleaned from such self-exploration introduces the vertical plane that contains knowing instead of remembered knowledge.

Isn't all of humanity given the key to exploring an inner world available to young and old alike? On this plane there are no favorites, no aristocracy, no hierarchy. Through a dialogue, the conversation on this plane is established between asking the question and waiting in silent expectation for an answer.

These are times when even objective realities have become illusory and alien to human beings. By questioning and listening to answers in silence, dialogue with the world beyond the sensory can unfold. Given that the tool of silent focus on an image results in answers flowing toward us as inspirations and intuitions, human understanding and acceptance of the vertical plane is not very far in the future.

Educators need to become clear that available resources and methods in the early twenty-first century are significant and enable the imaginative powers of children. After being held back for thousands of years, such resources from the heavens are again available to humankind.

The extraordinary human potential seen in our incarnating children (the Child Artist) can bring us not only the memories and experiences from pre-earthly existences and suprasensory realms, but can give humanity an opportunity to weave the potential for love and freedom as a leitmotiv throughout the history of civilization.

Plate 40: Focus

Alchemy as the First Science

For centuries the "language" of the alchemist was a silent speech. Through illustrations, the use of hieroglyphs, symbols, planetary and zodiacal references, and use of color designs and phonetics, an attempt was made to approach human senses with visual stimuli so that intuitive insights into nature and human connections could be awakened.

The body of knowledge called *alchemy* reaches at least five thousand years into antiquity, back to the Chinese culture of the Yellow King and the Sumerian culture of Ur. Cultural archives provide vivid descriptions of the mighty King Gilgamesh, who vanquished enemies and eternally befriended Enkidu–Eabani, who as a half-god was master of plant and animal kingdom. The body of science emerging in the Egyptian temples was secret wisdom called *kemy,* a term that may be found in hieroglyphs on Egyptian buildings and tombs. The actual meaning of this noun, as with most hieroglyphs, could be interpreted in more than one way. It is sufficient to mention three ways; the literal, the descriptive and flowery, and the secret and symbolic. In the literal sense *kemy* alludes to the black rich soil found around the Nile River. A deeper, more esoteric meaning understood and embraced by the initiated temple scholars: *"Something not seen—building blocks for the substances and objects that surround us."* The occult meaning must still elude us.

A thousand years later, with the rise of the cultures around the Mediterranean and a strong Saracen influence, the prefix *al* (as in Allah) was added. After 3,000 years of practice, study, and investigation, alchemy is now seen as a primitive form of science that nevertheless contributed to the development of modern chemistry and medicine. The prerequisite for students of alchemy was a combination of technical skill, obedience to the rule of secrecy, desire and curiosity for the unrevealed wonders of the universe, and a lifelong dedication to the projects investigated. The initiation of alchemy students included honing hidden capacities of vivid imaginations and listening in silence to inspirations of the gods, leading to intuitions that enrich human knowledge.

With the emergence of intellectual soul capacities, the curriculum was expanded; universities replaced temples for training, and the seven arts were inaugurated. This was a gain for young people, but also a loss for the inner capacities of imagination and the higher senses of inspiration and intuition. Initiation into knowledge and overextension of the thought process replaced the capacity for silence and listening to the gods conversing. Initiations were relegated to the religious orders, which instituted a separation of the sexes. Through the ages, few women were allowed to participate in studies of the seen or the unseen. Why?

During the pre-Christian era, all wisdom pertaining to nature phenomena, star wisdom, healing, and humanities was held within temple walls. It was secret and available only to appointed residents in those communities of scholars. The temples and the knowledge disclosed were under the protection of deities recognized by gender. The process of initiation could take years in the scholar's life, but once the initiate left a community it was strictly forbidden to divulge temple knowledge to the outside world. Socrates, as an initiate, was accused of teaching the young men of Athens, and he submitted to the resulting sentence of death by poison.

We have to wonder about the nature of these secret lessons. Most of what those teachers had to say is today part of the normal curricula of most elementary schools and can be found in Wikipedia and many other online sources. When young children are allowed to ponder the environment and the processes in nature that surround them, they can develop feelings of awe, and be stimulated by curiosity to experience the satisfaction of observing and understanding. Instead of relying on the memory and rote learning methods, children can develop through active participation in exchanges between teacher and student. This interaction is a platonic form of pedagogy in which the pupil can become the teacher, whereby we learn from one another regardless of age or position.

The many drawings made by a six-year-old—the "Child Artist"—demonstrate such a platonic exchange. The topic chosen by the young artist demonstrates his "knowing" of basic nature processes. The imaginations he shares reveal intimate familiarity with alchemical laws and introduce us to the advanced soul of a once-eminent mind, encouraging us to ask: Who are we meeting? Who teaches Us?

Processes in Nature

The expression of water under changing atmospheric conditions becomes a tool for grasping the processes of nature and the idea of metamorphosis of substance. When cold, the H_2O molecule changes to a crystal state. A snowflake, a brilliant star each uniquely formed with a six-arm configuration, falls from the sky in a fixed condition, embracing the Earth surface in a dusting of white salt. In the alchemist's laboratory, this was called the *salt process,* an activity of consolidation and crystal formation in a cold, dry environment.

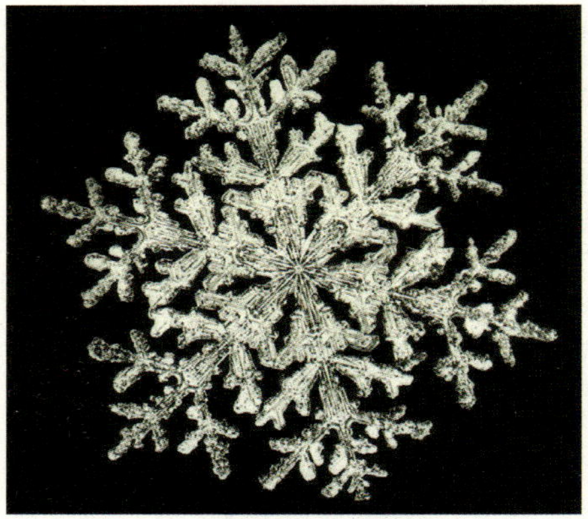

Plate 41: Snowflake

Ice is a solid, stone-like substance with the same molecule as water. The heat of the Sun and warmer weather melts the solid ice into water. The activity of the H_2O molecule changes to become livelier and the liquid state is introduced. Warmth brings H_2O into a solution, also referred to as the *solvent* process.

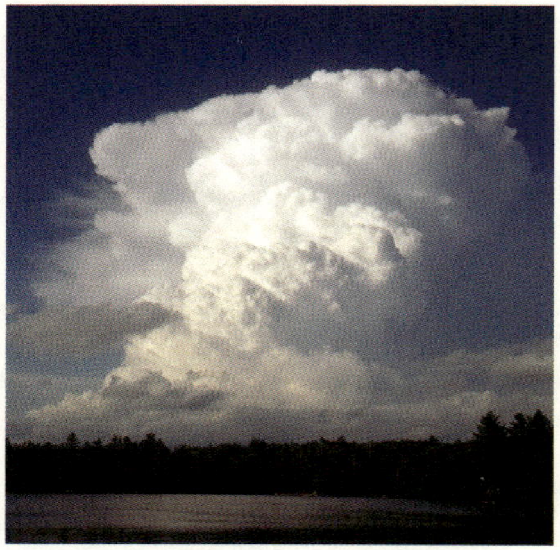

Plate 42: Cumulus cloud

In nature the atmosphere stimulates evaporation, the droplets disperse and move upward against the gravitational draw of the Earth to form clouds. A child can look up to the sky and be one with the bellowing towering white ac(cumulus) of water. In a kitchen, it is steam from the kettle; in nature it becomes fog or a cloud. In the state of fog, humidity penetrates throughout the atmosphere in a cloying repulsive fashion resembling the putrid sulfuric odor of a decaying product. When the dispersal process of nature takes place in a laboratory, it is called a *sulfur* process.

What do we find between these two poles of salt formation and the sulfur process of dispersion? In a laboratory this is the process

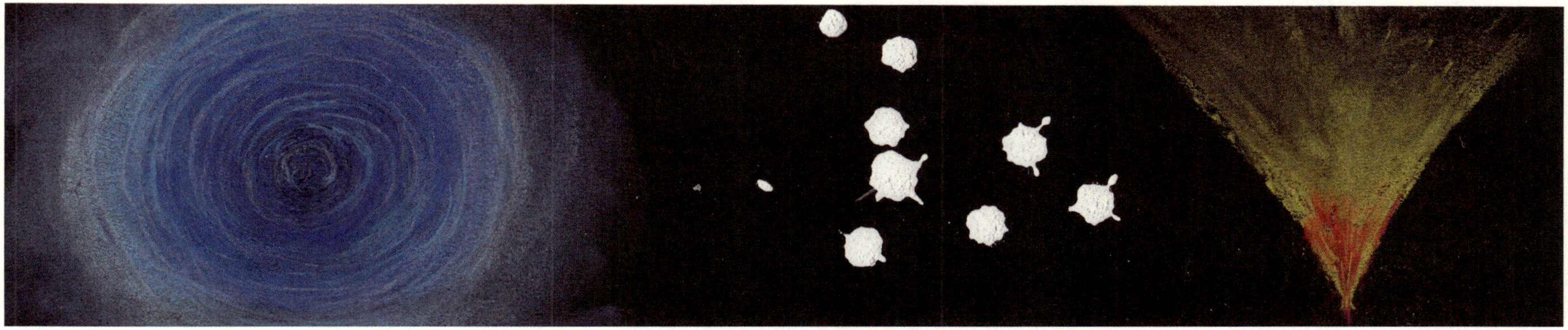

Plate 43: Salt mercury sulfur process

of droplet formation, and seen in nature as dew drops or rain. It is referred to as the *mercury* process.

Every child knows these words at an early age, and *snow, rain,* or *fog* form pictures in children's minds and become a part of their imagination. The processes of evaporation followed by condensation are procedures executed in the laboratory and practiced by alchemists to derive the substances they desire. Pupils become acquainted with the chemical characteristics of salt, mercury, and sulfur.

In the drawings of the Child Artist these basic nature processes are distinctly identified, indicating familiarity with the alchemical designations of salt formation, drop formation, and dispersion by way of gas or air. When questioning the mature Child Artist today on the significance of these images, there was no recognition of his own work. This proves to me that his process as Child Artist belongs to the unconscious, hidden memory—clearly one not connecting him to the stage of his life he is now experiencing. Although not penetrated into the Child Artist's consciousness, the exchange between the two of us is an example of platonic teaching, whereby I received and could interpret the mysterious, symbolic content of the drawings he presented. In further drawings, my choice of investigating alchemy in more depth will become very clear.

Alchemical Process	Salt	Mercury	Sulfur
Interpretation of Child Artist	Spiral	Eggs	Fountain
Associated Force	Centripetal	Balance	Centrifugal
Presentation in Nature	Crystal	Drop	Vapor
Phase	Solid	Liquid	Gas

The next step for the pupil in the temple schooling was to find the combination of these three processes of nature in one living form. This archetype is represented in the threefold structure of the plant—root, leaf, and flower. Where the root system is dominated by salt formation, the leaf system by the mercury process and the flower structure equating to the sulfur process, where it surrounds the reproductive organ of the plant to attract life forms helping in pollination. As a summary I have combined these three phenomena in nature, so that a distinct function can be appreciated.

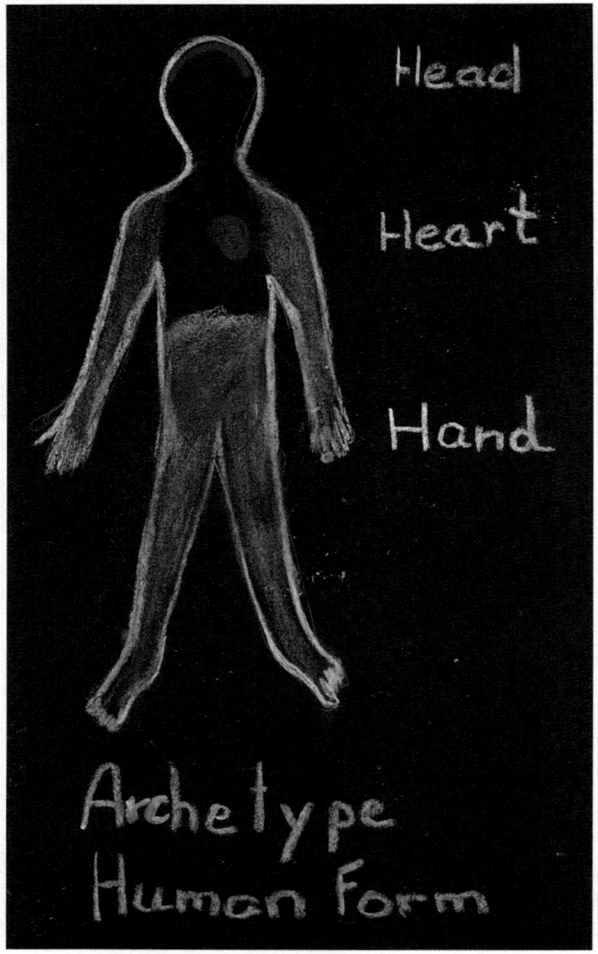

Plate 44: Archetype human form

Threefold Function in the Human Form

Liberty Hyde Bailey (1858–1954), a well-known American scholar, horticulturist, and author of *The Holy Earth* (1915), dedicated the last third of his life to social concerns of American youth and created the 4H movement, in which *Head, Heart, Hand* and *Health* indicated the need for striking a balance in the lives of teenagers. While living in Hillsdale (1972), I was asked to become a 4H leader of the local girls, setting examples in housekeeping, sewing, nutrition, and rhythm in daily life. Being fastidious, this was right up my alley, but I was able to keep up with that busy life for only one year. That was long enough though to encounter this respected scholar through his writings and to marvel at the wisdom of his ideas.

A balance of function in the three different parts of the body—the head for thinking, the heart for feeling, and the hand for will activity—brought home to me how important it is to distinguish the body's separation into three segments. Strangely enough, this scaffold has not been carried over, and the biography of Liberty Bailey is seldom mentioned today. The archetype of the human form can be seen in the threefold nature of head, heart, and hand, or the upside-down plant.

The content of the skull, the brain, is surrounded by the cerebral-spinal fluid and protected from gravity and sudden movements in a cocoon-like state. This part of human anatomy resembles the root system in the plant—kept in a state of darkness and protected from outside stimuli. The exchange of thought content becomes like a salt process.

The chest region containing the heart and the lungs is throughout life submitted to a steady, rhythmic four heartbeats to one breath of the lungs. The mercury process can be identified in the droplet structure of the alveoli and in the blood droplets of the circulation. Like the leaf distribution on the branch of the plant, the rhythmic quality is present throughout every aspect, imitating a breathing process of exhalation-inhalation for the exchange of oxygen and carbon.

Uncoordinated chaotic movements imbue all activity under the diaphragm. This process resembles a turbulent fomenting activity, with the production of sulfurous smelling gases in the gut. The sulfurous gesture is recognized in the plant in its flower formation. Through stimulation of the senses by the surrounding world (color or odor), the flower display brings the plant cycle to a conclusion. The reproductive nature of the plant uses the atomizing effect of sulfur to complete its procreation with the help of insects. The human limbs, the extremities enabling human movement, are incorporated into the lower system. Movement of the extremities in a newborn child is chaotic; human will forces develop toward a fluidity and grace only with training and the development of coordination. A unique signature is identifiable in the movement of a person.

Summary of Nature Processes and Correlations in the Human Being

Process	Salt	Mercury	Sulfur
Representation in Plant	Root	Leaf	Flower
Presentation in Nature	Snow Ice	Rain / Dew	Fog/Vapor
Representation in Human	Skull / Head	Heart / Lung	Hand / Gut
Seat of Soul Function	Think	Feel	Will

Three Kings

As a child between four and nine during World War II, much of my education was left to my own devices. Even at a young age, our homeschooling consisted of studying a phenomenon of our own choice for a day and reporting on it at the dinner table. Even an emotional observation counted as learning. There was tension on the streets as neighbors with yellow stars on their chest were deported. At night, with sirens blaring and the rumble of planes overhead, the three sibling children quickly descended into the dark stinky basement—waiting for what? Yet I had time to philosophize about the numbers—1, 2, 3, 4—and could look at them on paper, each shining with a different color and imbued by a distinct meaning. I could revel in this exploration, in the fact that, although just numbers, they had a deeper identity and significance for me. I loved the number three most of all because, although it represents three entities, I could imagine them having a fervent desire to melt into one again. Two was a split, but three representing the past, present, and future, all wrapped into one symbol. How could I have known then that a boy, the same age that I was then, would introduce me after fifty-six years with a new challenge to this mysterious thrice/one symbol?

It was surprising when the Child Artist handed me this picture I titled "The Initiation of the Three Kings" (refer plate 20). Careful examination introduces us to two sources of enlightenment for the three crowned figures being initiated. First the earthly source in the form of the fountain. This we previously introduced as the source of mercurial powers personifying the quality of life through the function of breathing. On Earth the home of life is the "living" water contained in all life forms. The three figures all wearing a crown, share the two overflowing sources, but with careful observation I discern a moving quality in this picture.

Let's examine the heavenly body in the left corner. "Oh, that is the Sun!" I say. But look carefully, this orb, radiating warmth (red) and light (yellow), is hollow and filled with a being. The distribution of the three figures is uneven; under the bestowing orb, two of the figures are tardy. One figure has "moved on" and has received "blessing" from the Earth—the fountain of living water springing from the depths. This drawing does convey movement, the experience of the figures on a "spiritual" path from left to right while experiencing or inundated so to say with sources of Warmth, Light from above and Life from the Earth center. This drawing represents a ceremony enacted for perhaps only one person—not just once but three times. Who are the Three Kings? Could the three figures represent one being who thrice repeats a blessed immersion into life vouchsafed by earthly wisdoms?

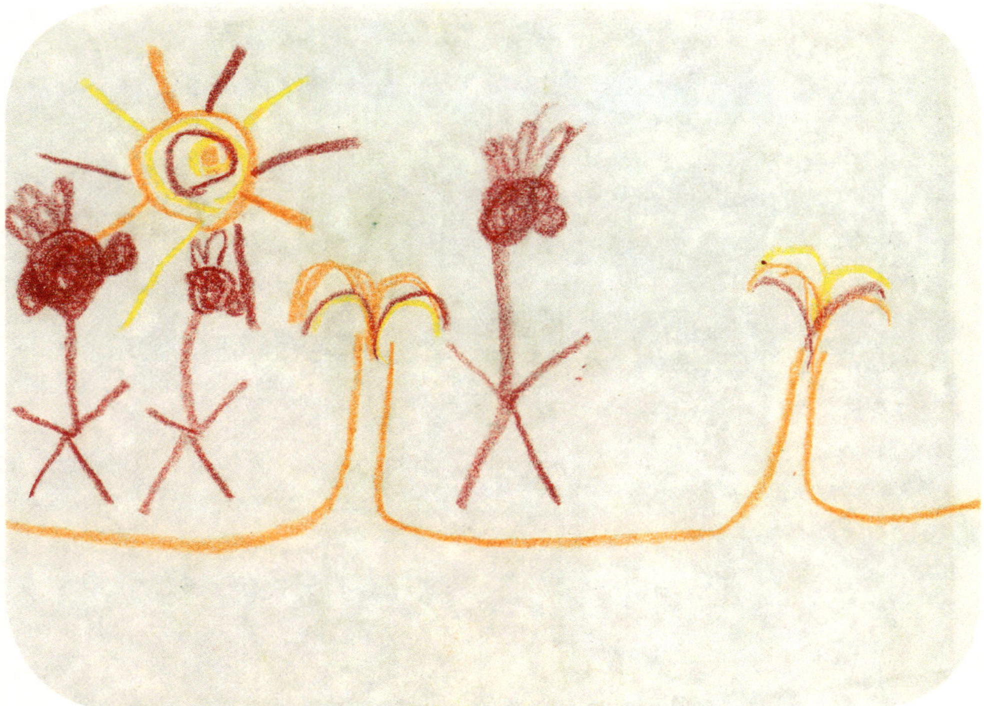

Plate 45: Three Kings (reproduced)

The re-introduction of Three Kings as the lofty Hermes Trismegistus together with the opportunity to reconsider his postulates in the form of The Tabula Smaragdina becomes a new imagination that combines the work of the Master with one of his pupils, the Child Artist. The teachings in the Tabula draw attention to the physical incarnation of the human being in a step wise construction of the embryonic body. He conveys the magnitude of **The One** being the human embryonic presence. He continues to mention the contributions of the four cosmic regions (*sun, moon, air, and earth*), that augment (perfuse) the solid constitution derived from the reproductive cells of the parents. He declares himself as the master of knowing these reproductive processes with unassailing certainty.

In the Child Artist we discover two illustrations that lead us into the imaginative world of past knowing. First the wonderful initiation of the Three Kings that acquaints us with the Tabula Smaragdina. Second the one truthful illustration involving the stages in embryonic development. These are the stepping stones on which I can build my hypothesis of the wonders of **The One** and thereby awaken also in my own biography the authenticity and hopeful future.

Revisiting the emerald tablet becomes the goal in this biography. Together with the illustrations of the Child Artist, I am able to explore a meaningful discussion of the postulates in section E (ey), which includes drawings of embryological forms.

Alchemical Equipment

The pictures of the Child Artist continues to take us on a tour. The secret codes and drawings he shares are filled with riddles and conceal truths. For the student and interpreter the challenge remains in how far we have understood the language. In visiting the "master" in his schooling of Alchemy he was generous to share indications of equipment used in the laboratory of old. The outstanding example is the Green Truck drawing for which we found an excellent comparative in Roobs that we demonstrate here.

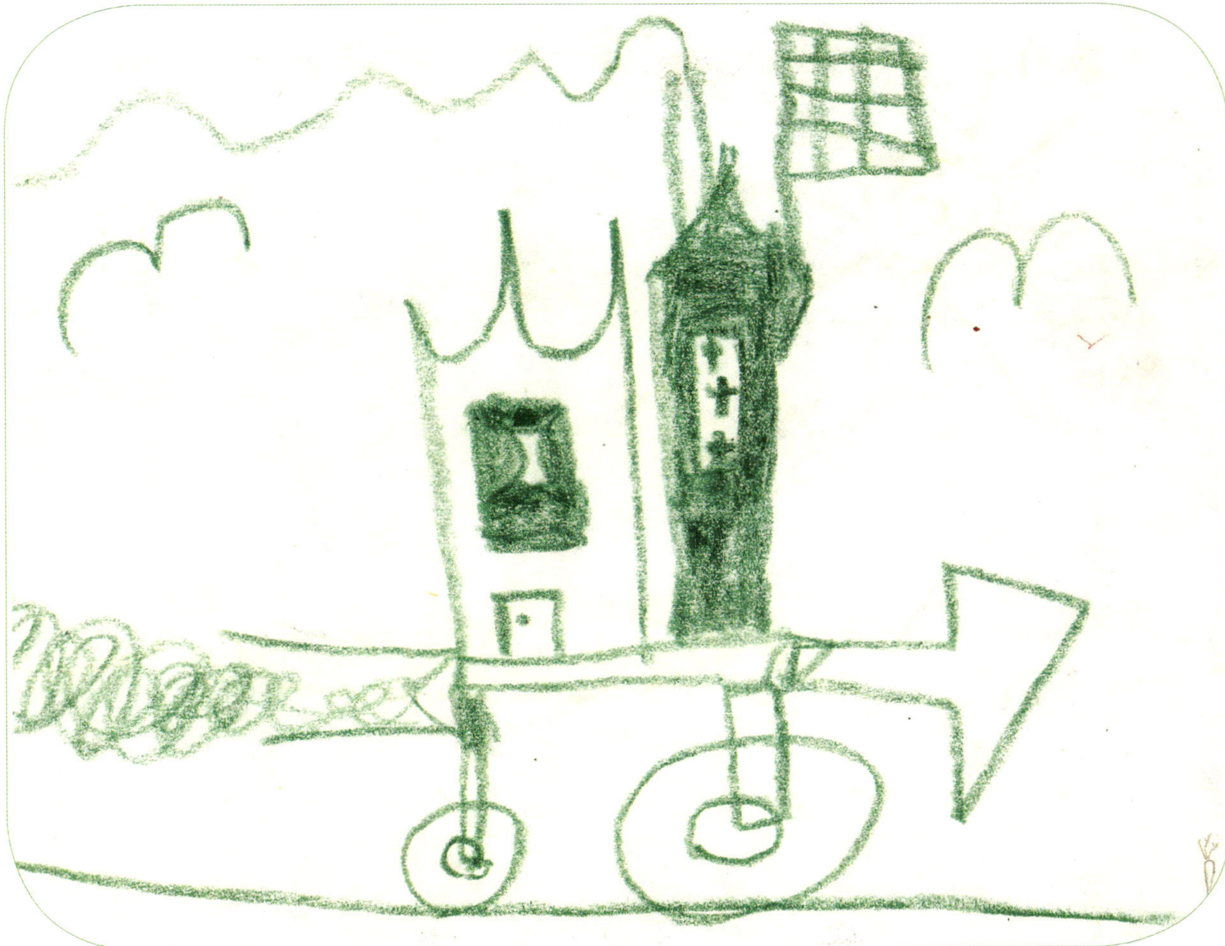

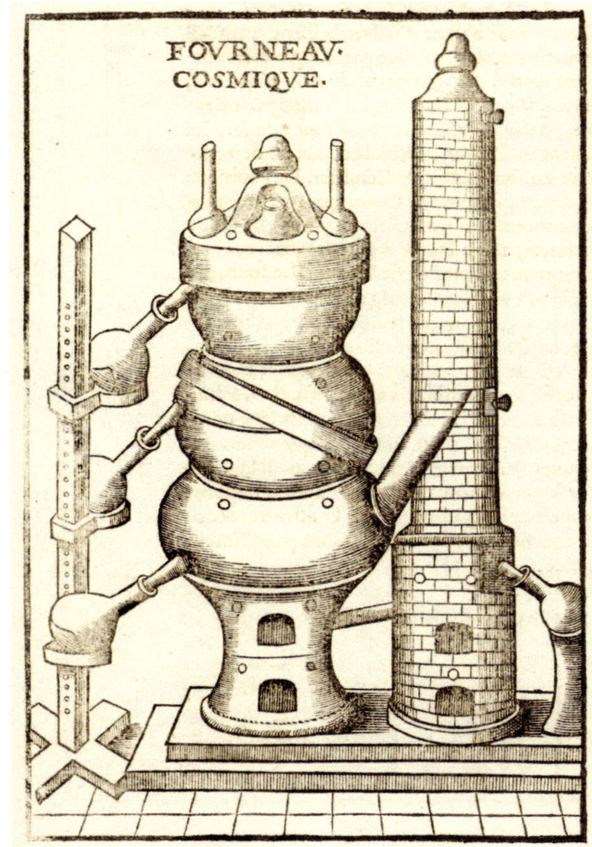

Plate 46: Reproduction of Green Truck as comparison to alchemical equipment

The Path of Initiation for the Alchemist

Considering, thousands of years that the discipline of Hermetic science or Alchemy influenced learned men and women, I have become convinced that the Gnostic myths played a definitive role in soul development of many of these students. This myth will play a role in the Genesis story that will unfold in the next section when both the biblical Genesis and embryogenesis is illuminated. For alchemical students on a path of initiation, elements of dark matter in their own soul life needed to be expunged, undergo sublimation, and transformed into *lapis,* to return into the paradisiacal primordial state. Finding the correct pathway was a chief concern and this secret was protected throughout the ages by code names, symbols, and illustrations. Obviously a guide or master was still needed. The journey required a passing through the outermost circle of the underworld, a world filled with monsters and beastly creatures, a world so frightening that only through conjuring up courage and the help of the divine world, was the student enabled to complete his task. Enlightenment does not come without hurdles.

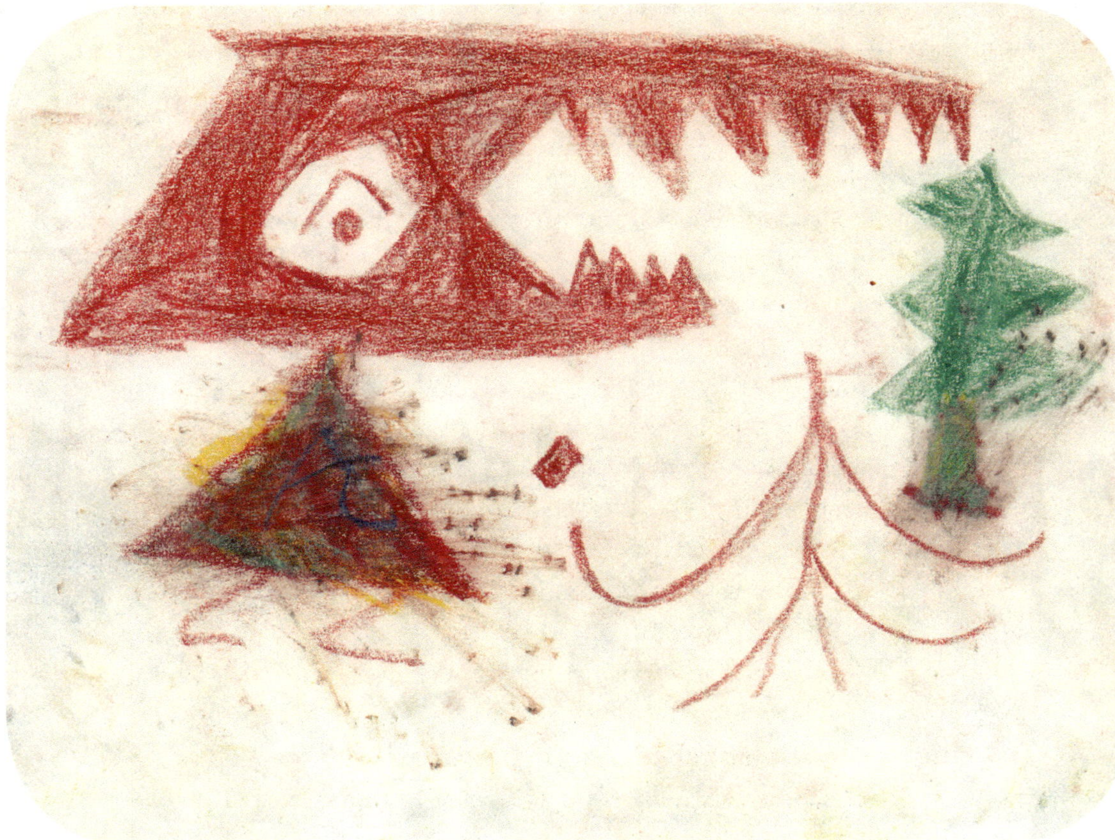

Plate 47: Return of the Devouring Monster

The Monster (ref. plate 9) presented in the Gallery, calls for a conclusion of the Child Artist's work. Like a mythical Seth, this fierce monster devours all that is alive and in its wake leaves chaos and destruction. Hope and courage are the two contributions attained by the graduate and the promise of a meaningful future for Earth and humanity.

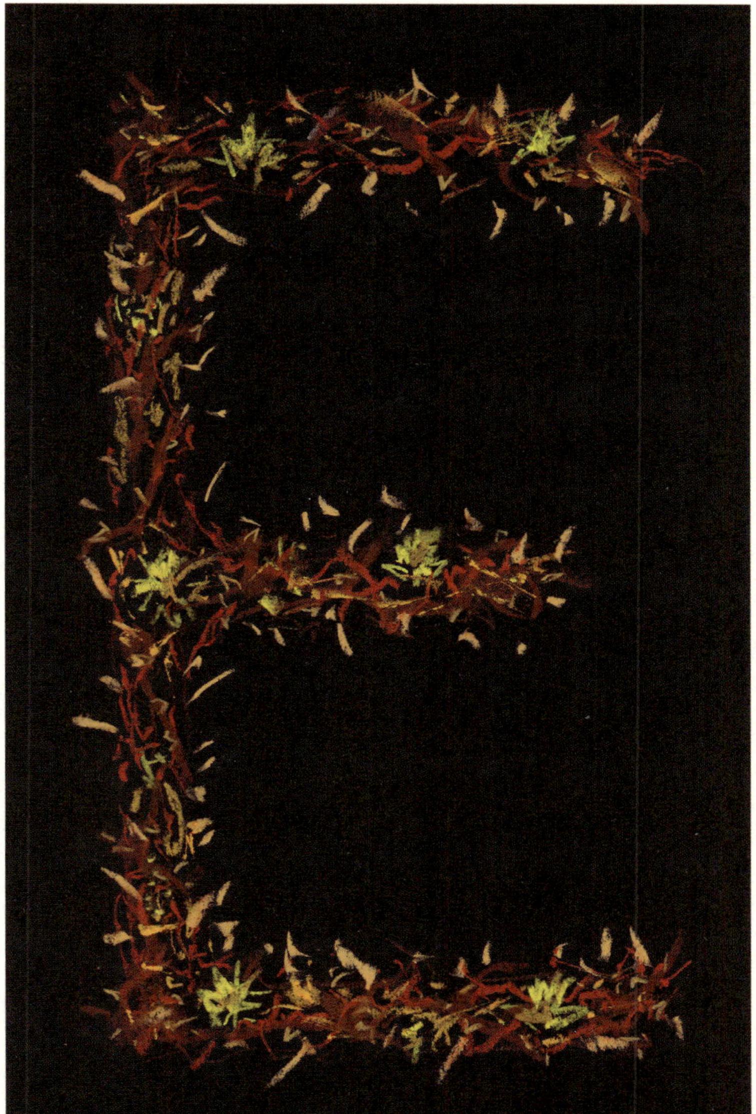

Plate 48: Sound E as depiction

Sound E

In this chapter we meet a gesture that lives in a duality of a short staccato followed by an uninterrupted, longer, transformed circular movement. Throughout space the short exclamation of E (ey) forcefully interferes with the primary centrifugal flowing of the A (ah) gesture. This crossing brings the possibility of change in existing dynamic flow. Together with the perseverance in the turbulence and seeming chaos created during this confrontation is the experience of a crossover. Not in a collision but a sensitive rising in awareness of another force. The short staccato E (ey) begins to establish boundaries, moments of holding the outward flow at bay introducing possibilities for something new to be created. Becoming aware, creating a consideration for the new or other, sensitivity to what is in the backspace, and establishing a duality are all part of this energy. Like a pendulum, the direction of flow is arrested after the first exuberant extension.

Including this vowel E (ay) vocabulary *awakens* the human being to action or defense. Crossing the limbs in front of the body is a defensive act toward what comes toward us from the periphery.

A counter movement now is introduced and the two opposite forces meet while the sound E (ey) is heard. The being of E (ey) with swift lightness, raised arms crossed over, warding off the overwhelming flow of forward movement. NAY—no further, stop! In nature we find the same gesture when a rapid flowing stream is interrupted with a stone or tree branch. Turbulence creates small vortexes; a circular dynamic becomes the origin for a new impulse.

In the recognition of a threefold human being (body, soul, and spirit) it follows that the creation takes place in the beginning of things (Genesis).

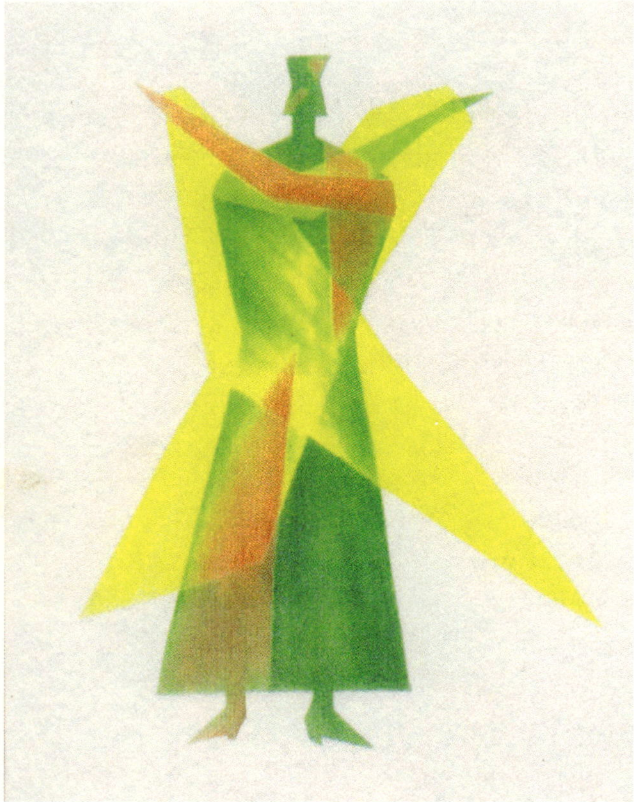

Plate 49: Eurythmy gesture of E

The soul as an organ housed in the physical body, finds its origin through Gaya undergoing a descent into darkness.

In the sounding of A(ah) throughout space a new impulse arises. It is the E (ey) sound thwarting the unobstructed forward flowing impulse of beginnings. It becomes the place for examining the incarnating process. First the human being, **The One**, imbued with spirit, descends from the outer reaches of the celestial spheres with a relationship to the Gaya, who as God-Creator, reaches out (over) from beyond other dimensions. **The One** incarnating into the world of solidity by descending into the parental cells of reproduction reveals threefold merging—father, mother, and cosmic visitor—is introduced by the knowledge of embryogenesis. Two dynamics occur, one macrocosmic (the human spirit) coming from outer spaces, the other microcosmic (embryo) unfolding in the most intimate space of human anatomy, the pelvis; yet each with a similar reaction to the symphonic music of the spheres, the vowel sounds.

The vibration of the distinct vowel sounds ring through the space. This journey can best be experienced within the body, if the reader can evoke the imagination with the voice sounding the vowels as I have demonstrated. Taking ourselves through the vowel sounds A-E-I-O-U in bodily expression and pronunciation one experiences a possibility of deeper penetration correlating with increased density. Ending with the U sound, we experience a solid pillar, immovable upright supporting all contained within—sustainable and separate from Earth.

History of the Gnostic Myth

Throughout the ages, all the cultures of the East, West, South, and North had, as a social foundation, a creative myth in which the Gods descended, fructified the Earth, and left human beings to their own devices. Knowledge belonging to supraearthly dimensions, the existence of creative gods, and the placement of the human being into the order of creation are all assigned to the spiritual aspect of humanity. We can find such stories in the older scriptures of Tibet, India, Persia, and the Talmud and Gnostic books of the Jewish people. The inheritance of this material is vouchsafed to all human beings regardless of their orientation and will be a source for the recognition of the power of **The One**. It becomes clear that human beings are the only spiritual entities to pursue a path into matter. The gaze of multiple Gods follows us with the creator god Gaya leading us down into ever increasing density. We experience this imaginative picture as a powerful reminder that loneliness will be felt if the "I" is cut off from the reality of existing gods. These beings do have a vital interest in human individuality.

Out of this Gnostic myth, with Gaya as the mother to lead humanity toward new existence, an electrifying story unfolds. Her descent out of the Godhead is not in silence but with the background of the music of the spheres, the cosmic ringing of the vowels, all creative forces influencing the process of becoming. It is not given to humanity to abide by; it becomes a subjective imagination that can fit in each human being's personal confession of faith (The Credo).

Humans as created light-beings are assigned a place in creation as the tenth hierarchy. They are described as descending into the dark cold prison of solidity that is created by Gaya. In the struggle for release and return to the Father God they are assigned to generate Love and Freedom as an investment for the entire created world. In this process of evolution, creative sound experienced as a vibrational music or word, influences the travelers. The sounding of the vowels will continue to be an experience in the process of solidification.

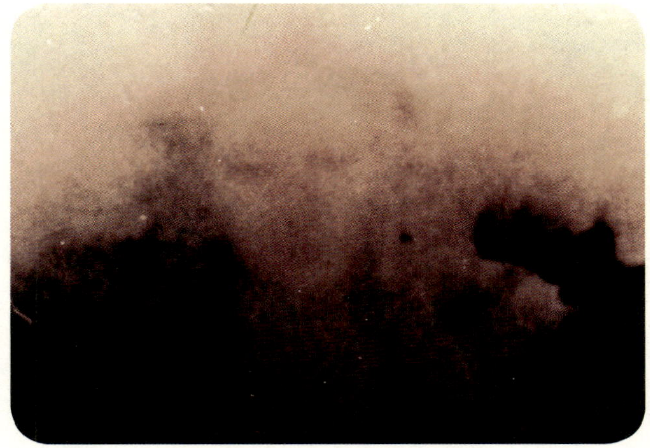

Plate 50: Image of Sophia

It can also be imagined that this being, in her descent, escorts and protects the human sparks in their becoming. An imagination of how the step-wise birth of the soul occurs, we can find in the powerful myth of Gaya, also known to us as the Sophia relating to the planetary bodies (solar system). She created the Earth and remains on the level of our existence as a pure refined presence still incorporated in all of living matter. Although some of humanity is not aware, **SHE IS WITH AND IN US**. In her evolution she is born anew as unsoiled human nature. She is seen in the suprasensory experiences of pure souls, such as children. She will communicate with those human beings whose childlike existence

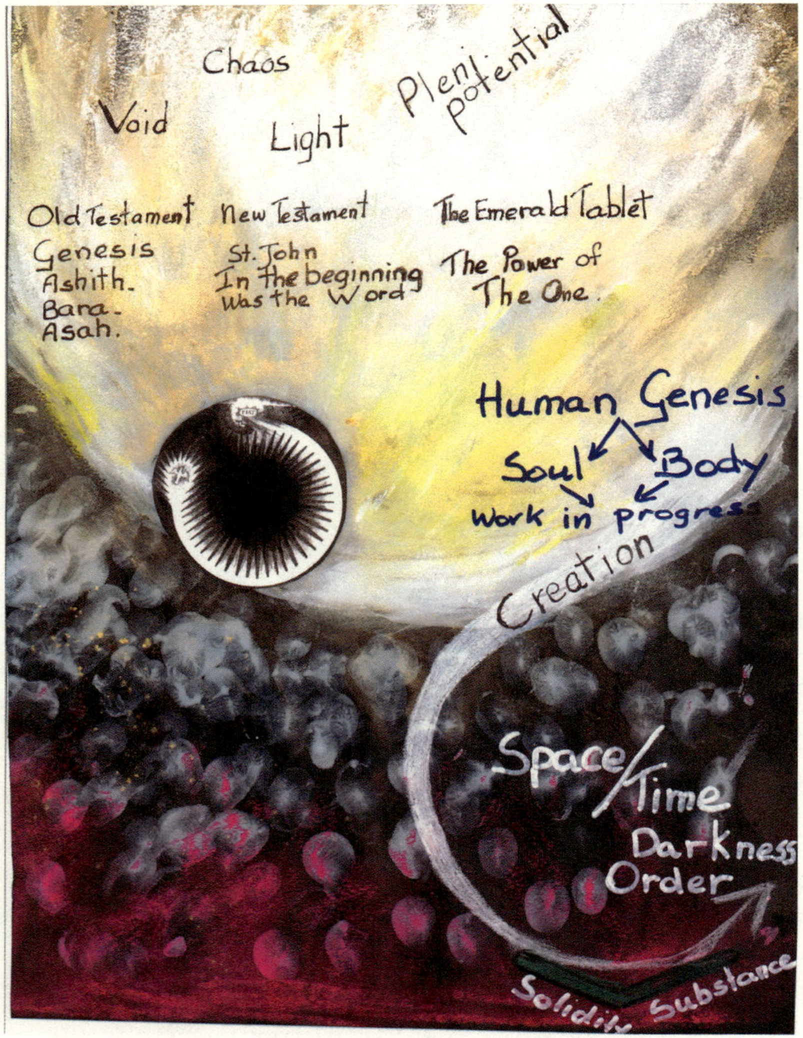

Plate 51: Soul genesis

can endure her presence (plate 23). Goethe (*Faust*) names her the eternal Feminine redeeming the fallen human being.

The presence on Earth of millions of individualities, reflecting their uniqueness in the protein scaffolding they carry, is in itself a wondrous cosmic occurrence to be contemplated. The individuality, introduced as **The One,** through the work in the Emerald Tablets, has an intimate relationship to this feminine celestial being.

The creative process one witnesses in the evolution and maturation of the human soul and physicality will be considered. Imagination affords us the sharing of the Gnostic creation myth of Gaya, who here is identified as the "SOUL of HUMAN"

This is the pluripotent moment of Gaya setting out of the heavens. The Bible (Gen. 1:2) describes the darkness referring to an immaterial existence as void and chaos. This nothingness referred to in the Hebrew original text was without time or space. It could be recognized in a condition of pure intense light. Many possibilities did it hold, chaos seethed, new potentials were constantly emerging. Divine beings worked as one, they obeyed the rules of a grand being referred to as *THE FATHER GOD*. IT existed as a radiation of pure love. Through ITS presence all was made possible. Without ITS presence nothing was made. Humanity was the latest creation, behind the nine hierarchies already ruling and working throughout the heavens as creators of worlds.

The building of the physical body is relegated to **The One** and becomes the story of embryogenesis. Dimensions of time and space are the accouterments of the earthly physicality dived into by **The One** at the moment of merger in the act of fertilization.

I give to you the beautiful myth of the Gaya (*Gaia*), Sophia captured in a poem by an Estonian female, her Mother God stepping from the highest and loftiest abode and dwelling after the fiat is consented to by the Father God. When pure light meets darkness or absence of light, red is created.

Gaia Sophia
On foot I had to walk through the solar systems,
Before I found the first thread of my red dress.
Already I sense myself.
Somewhere in space hangs my heart,
Sparks fly from it, shaking the air,
To other reckless hearts.

—**Stina Katchadourian**

Soul Genesis

To understand the existence of a soul, a personality, and an individuality dwelling in the same earthly body, makes us question our own uniqueness and signature. What is the story of my beginning? Can the manifestation of the personality, changing with different incarnations, make a claim in developing sense and soul organs with renewed improvement? In the last greeting of a dying Cherokee, the inculcated wish for *a better life the next time*, is expressed.

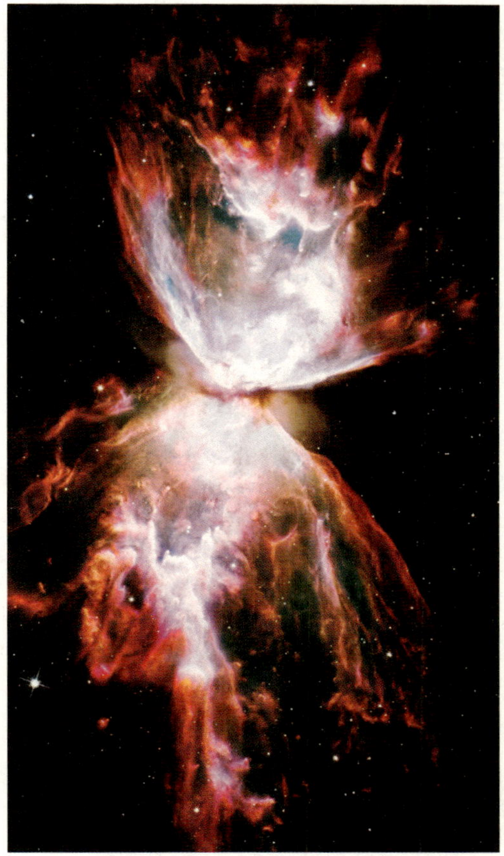

Plate 52: NASA nebula

First one must acknowledge that the Sophia escorts and protects **The One** from the state of A (ah). **The One** experiences safe passage through the celestial spheres ending with its incarnation in form—the process of conception. At this crossing, the stream of the A (ah) becomes turbulent, fluctuating and finally breaking down into individual drops cut off from the stream. Where the A (ah) is timeless the introduction of flowing time is a result of this drop formation. On Earth the individual exists in time.

The "I" or soul experience of the human being is steeped in time. Memories are the cornerstone of the soul experience. We gather sense perception of a lifetime granted to us through the natural world. This world being our Earth, so beautifully organized and maintained by the Mother Sophia.

The human's organ of soul comes under the purview of our cosmic mother (referred to as MAYA by Rudolf Steiner) and the poignant meditation in the Misraim service reminds all of **The Ones** that she will continue to present herself through the HUMAN SOUL.

If you approach me with true desire for knowledge
I shall be with you.
I am the germ and the source of your visible world,
I am the sum of the light in which your soul lives
I am she who rules in space,
I am she who creates the cycles of time,
Fire, Air, Light, Water, and Earth obey me.
Perceive me as the immaterial origin of all matter
And, as I have no husband on Earth,
call me therefor "Maya."

— **Rudolf Steiner**
(*"Freemasonry" and Ritual Work,* p. 244)

Each human spark created received an assignment: "As individualities they would descend into the darkness, and become the first hierarchy creating and subsequently penetrating solid substance" (Myth of Creation). Solid substance means the world of molecules. This dense material is to serve as the garment of **The One**, becoming home to the human being and reenacted until free from the wheel of repetitive life karma. Bondage and darkness is assigned to humanity stimulating the desire for freedom and light. Humanity, as the tenth hierarchy, was given the task to develop a soul disposition toward LOVE and FREEDOM. This would be an original contribution to benefit all of creation.

Through the descent of the divine Gaya, humanity became endowed with the sense organ of soul and the "I" organization, three distinct aspects in the conscious human being. These aspects—the soul in its capacity to Love and Hate, the sense organs of which at this time only five are familiar to us, and the "I"-organization also identified as the Self who observes conscious activity and inserts the processes of thinking, feeling and will—are gifts of the Sophia, that divine being who accompanied us on the descending journey into darkness.

Let us repeat again the journey of the Gaya and find the correlation between the soul and the physical body of **The One** in the following lines. With the A(ah) resounding space opens, and Gaya clothed in a luminous white garment, steps out of the world of Heaven. Millions of light sparks (human spirits) follow her passionate descent, awaiting birthing into dark realms. While hearing the A(ah) throughout cosmic space, the light meets dark, creating the color red. Gaia's garment flows in waves and frills like the Aurora high over the poles, high above the atmosphere, undulating. So far—So close! Overwhelmed with magnificence and familiarity, humans as sublime light sparks sense and wait. The first acquisition in this birthing process is that what is sensed by Gaya, the color of red. This is awakening of the soul through sense. A stage in consciousness is where the human "I" lives in its newly achieved sense perception of color and sound. The "I" embodies sense perception as the first step in creation. The gesture is one of overflowing, perpetual motion, tumbling into dark, creating red in its wake. The human "I" dives into existence and red blood will become its organ. This becomes the imprint for the "I" (individuality) and can also referred to as destiny.

In our creation myth Gaya is freed from her exsanguination. She adjusts, and human soul is freed from bondage to the senses of only vision and hearing.

Evolution of the Soul-Psyche

In the imaginary breathing-out ("I" am not) followed by breathing in ("I" am), the reality of imprisonment within the boundaries of a physical existence is discovered. Spirit freedom is sacrificed when polarities, with the choices they offer, are introduced in bodily formation. The soul receives within its boundary the polarity of Love–Hate, the capacity for desire or rejection. The body development (embryogenesis) creates boundaries adhered to by the Soul.

In the embryo the sequence of development is first red blood cell formation, capillaries of the periphery, smaller and larger venous system, large veins, the heart. This duct system is assigned to contain the organ of blood that is the seat of the "I." **The One** has found its place from which to rule the embryo-genetic development. This circulatory organ becomes responsible for the delivery of the blood throughout the physical body. The heart itself functions as a sense

Physical Incarnation—Soma

The human "I" bathes in the red color, the color of Gaia's garment.
This becomes the color of the human blood formed in the embryo.
Blood cells move from the periphery toward the center (centripetal).
The "I"-organization claims the blood cell formation, and with a rhythmic pendulum movement establishes the circulation.
In the Embryo a new stage is entered.
Fluid flowing from the periphery into the center, centripetal coming abruptly to rest at the center.
This becomes a place where mingling of air and liquid is possible.
A new creative possibility is added, that of foam formation.
Fluid penetrated with air makes bubbles, like the interruption of liquid flow, creating foam. Formation of alveoli in the lung and the globules in the glandular organs are an outcome of this dynamic process.
The lung organ makes it possible for the "I"-organization to experience the pulsing and rhythm, at that point where streaming of blood and potential flowing of air intertwine.
Through the awareness of the space-behind created in the sound E(ey) the first organ is created: that of the heart.
The embryonic task, under the vowel sounding is completed when a crossover between two tubular structures, later designated as venous and arterial streaming, takes place. The heart becomes a hollow space.
The two organs in the chest region, heart and lung, become the organs expressing feeling. The soul experiences feeling through pulses and rhythms—the intersecting flow of blood with flowing air.

organ, interrupting the blood flow and listening to information from both the upper and lower poles of the body. The blood as a fluid organ is recognized as the bearer of the most sacred aspect of the human being, the "I," the human soul. Its expression is through the rhythm of the pulsing heart with respiration, in the contraction and relaxation of peripheral capillaries of the skin. The autonomous nervous system becomes the servant, when we blush or pale in soulful meeting with "the other."

There are two illustrations of the Child Artist I want to bring to your attention. Both are fragments out of the large Plate no 3 the drawing of the heart (plate 20) and Plate no 21 the drawing of the Sun (plate 22) respectively. Of interest is the content we can extract out of both drawings when we enlarge the representations. The heart drawn with four colors has a winged being in yellow in the center. Also with the Sun picture we notice a window with a distinct face looking down upon the scenario of the Three Kings. The heart ruled by the Sun, plays a prominent role in the evolution of the human being. We can ask the child: "Where is your soul?" and it will place its hand on the left side of the chest where the heart pulsates.

The Eastern Medicine imagination of the heart function is described in the following meditation.

It governs the Blood
It controls the blood vessels
It manifests in the completion
It houses the Shen
It opens the tongue
It controls sweat

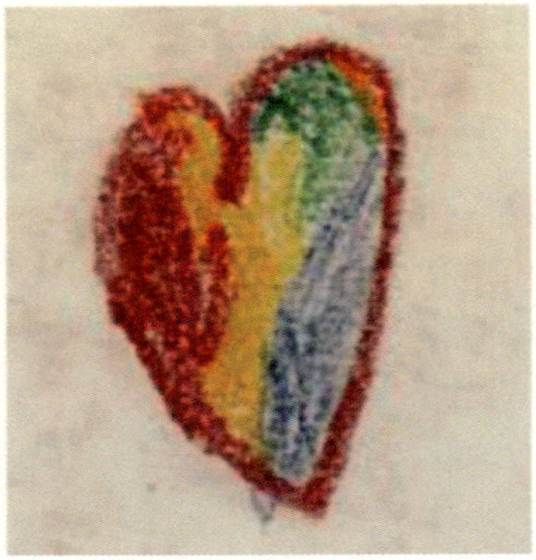

Plate 53: Heart (reproduced)

One may appropriately ask here: "Is the heart a pump"?

An independence of soul is established once the developing embryonic organ can imbibe light and warmth. Once the individuation takes place the interior space fills with blood (the seat of the soul), establishing a rapid and expansive growth pattern of tissue. **The One's** incarnation phenomenon becomes the individuation process resulting in a sole identity. Once in a state of mature adulthood the strength of blood assists in the struggle for a virtuous existence. **The One** has been tasked for its incarnation on Earth and is able to express itself through both the soul and the physical body. **The One** in its personification on Earth, observes, corrects, encourages, tutors, and loves its earthly counterpart with utmost endurance and patience. The "I" is present in the expression of the faculties, both in body and soul, with which all humans are endowed. While dwelling on Earth a strong "I" foremost expresses soul qualities of balance between the capacities of focused thinking, feelings as expressed in emotions, and control of the will. Its physical expression, endurance, and perseverance throughout physical hardships or failures are recognizable.

Gaya created for humanity a solar system of planetary bodies in which the Sun becomes the pivotal life-imbuing central sphere (star). Earth has soul, created as the habitat for life, becomes the body of the Gaya who we identify as a living entity, Sophia. Through Her creative impact, the body of the human is constituted out of forces from all the planets and contributes to its constitution (astral body). The eternal feminine represents humanity in its wholeness. It is the Sophia intertwined with the human being (*Anthropo-Sophia*) whose wisdom culminates in the highest spiritual aspect—the wondrous physical living body. It can be called "The Symphony of the Created World."

Embryogenesis: Incarnation of The One

Embryology as a science allows us to examine the day-to-day incarnating process of the individual human being. In science it represents the meeting of the two reproductive cells during fertilization and its development. It does not include the incarnation of the human spiritual spark at the moment of the cell merger. It is through the work of the Child Artist that our consciousness of this process is awakened. Interpretation of the Child Artist's drawings becomes an essential part in considering the formative force of **The One**.

Natural science teaches that the dynamics of the male and female reproductive cells is simply represented in a merger of two cells becoming one. By introducing a new possibility derived out of the combined works of the Child Artist, the gnostic mythical story of Gaya bringing humanity into fulfillment of incarnating "in the flesh" and the highly respected Initiate of Alchemy Hermes Trismegistus and his writing of the *Tabula Smaragdina* or the Emerald Tablet, a new story for the incarnating human being can unfold and be contemplated.

Still in the dynamics of the Ah flow the sojourn of the Spirit from the higher regions is completed. It needs to be acknowledged that the element of time is negligible because the genesis aspect is beyond the dimensions of time.

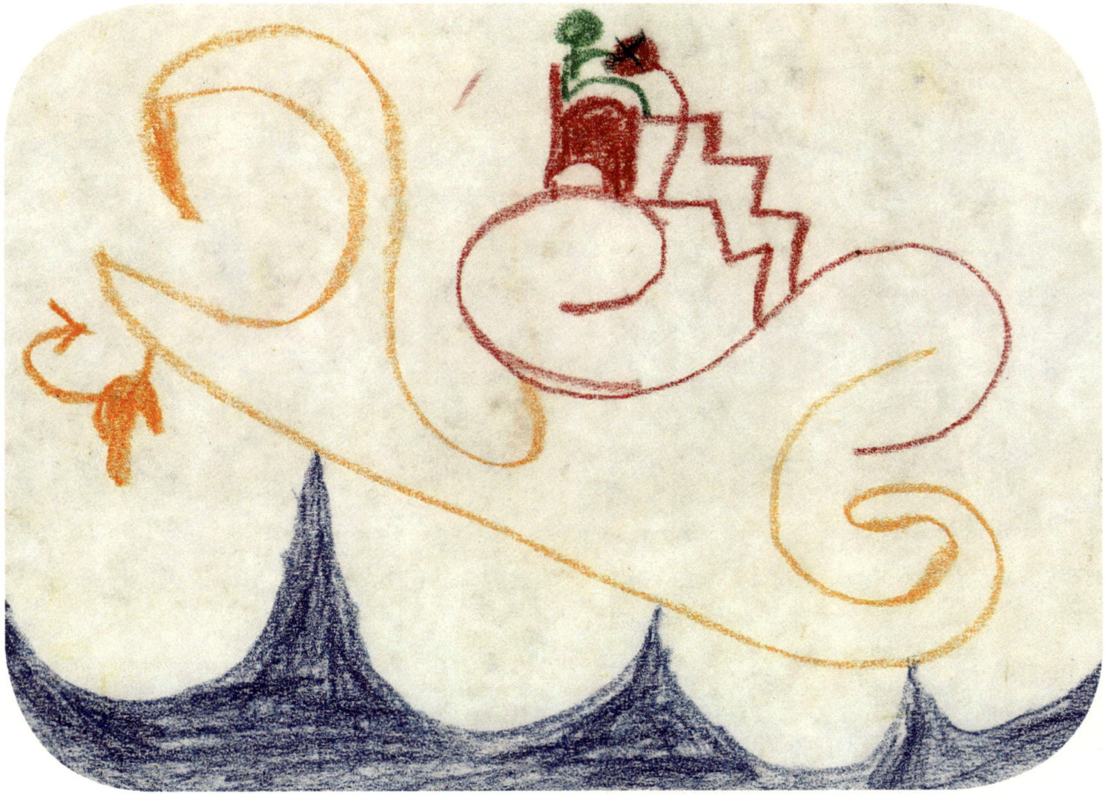

Plate 54: Cosmic sled on choppy waters (reproduced)

The descent of **The One** from cosmic regions is eloquently presented in three pictures by the Child Artist. They represent a space journey between the Sun and the Earth. In the first picture (plate 12) the origin of **The One** is eluded to when the artist includes the Sun in the left-hand corner. The Sun and Moon, represented as the fountain symbol, become the sustainable sources of warmth, light, and life that the existence on Earth will incorporate. The "ship" available to him is fitted out with a perfect round cosmic sail, and an intricate rudder system. The cabin is closed designating the cosmic being as a passive passenger. A chaotic plasmatic presence is situated on the front bow (ref. plate 12).

A totally different impression is created with the illustration titled the cosmic chariot (plate 13) reproduced below. Studying this glorious representation one is drawn into the movement of the vehicle downward, the choppy waves beneath, and the masterful command the captain asserts from way above. The seat is elevated like a throne, the rudder is solidly connected to all the limbs, and for The One there is only one way... onward! The steering mechanism is again an important accouterment to the drawing and it tells us a story of unwavering intentionality.

Moments before the penetration into solidity, at the time of fertilization, **The One** reflects the uncertainty it experiences (preview). The enormity of the earthly task, facing loneliness, deprived of spirit sensing, all of this could overwhelm, if it was not for the angelic guardian being standing right next to the small figure, embracing the traveler with a long arm of protection.

Now the sail becomes like angel wings as a reminder that return is still possible? Around the incarnating being earthly life forces find expression in multiple birds flying around the boat. The heart shaped structures symbolically represent **The One's** capacity for love toward all it meets. There is a disconnection (earphones?) to

Incarnation is the descent of a sentient being from outer cosmic regions. During the merger or material manifestation of this force, whose original nature is immaterial, the conception or birth is completed. —***Wikipedia***

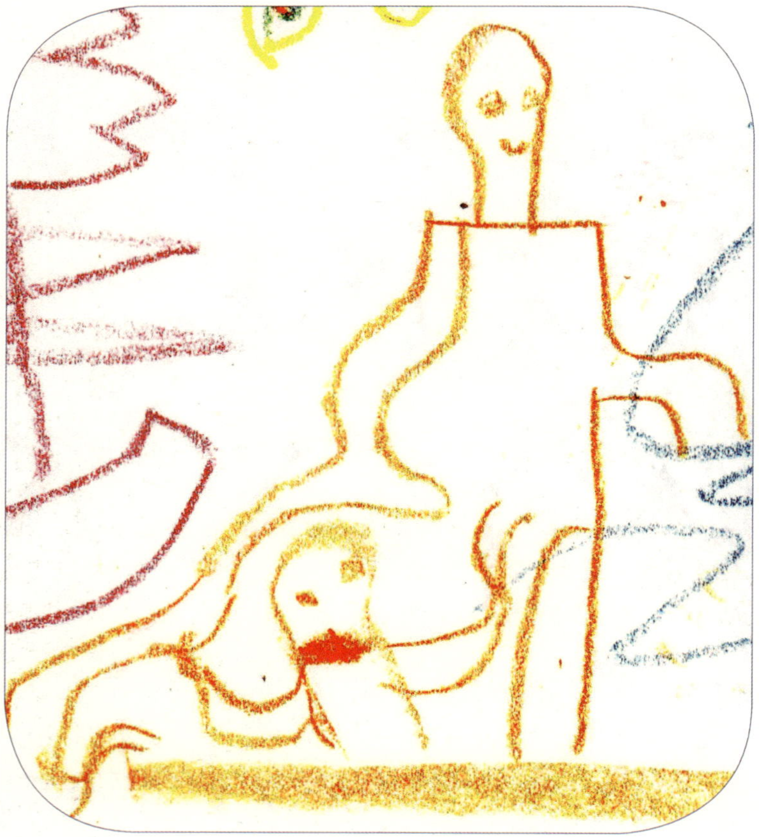

Plate 55: The Guardian (fragment)

the always-available cosmic musical succor. During the meeting on the horizontal plane a guardian or guide accompanies the enthusiastic traveler.

The interpretations of these symbolic illustrations are subjective and an imaginative freedom is practiced owing to our limitations in grasping the suprasensory. Naming the incarnating **One** *Spirit* or *individuality* is irrelevant. The process of incarnation is recognized in the following definition (see the comment from Wikipedia above left).

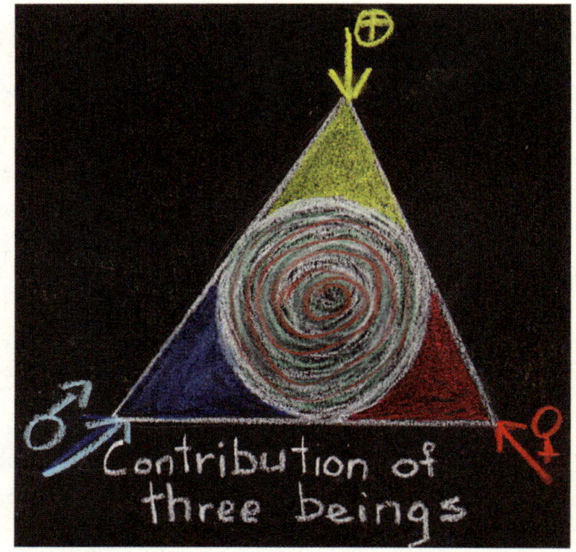

Plate 56: Contributions of three beings

Incarnation and conception occur under an evolutionary dynamic in the sound of the E (ey). During and after the dynamic two streams crossing, new beginnings are created. The dimension of time, foreign to spirit is introduced. The male and female gametes are prepared long before the fertilization to be haploid in chromosomes. The splitting of chromosomes from the natural number of forty-six to only twenty-three in both gametes is a necessary precursory step to the fertilization process. Of note is the amazing fact that each of these gametes contains unique protein configurations (snowflake).

This same gesture is observed in the spirit-being just before the sperm penetration of the ovum. While hovering over the parental

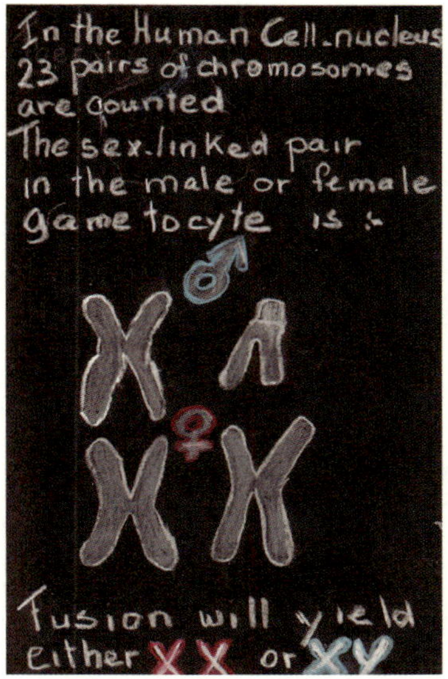

Plate 57: Gender chromosomes

gamete cells a division into two streams or forces responsible for different activities in the development of the embryo is enacted. The first part spirit-germ connects with the physical body and is instrumental in determining form and shape. The second part spirit-body will individualize the embryo.

One can imagine that the spirit-germ chooses one particular sperm cell and directs that parental donor to penetrate the mother cell. Keep in mind that the male gamete assigns gender. The incarnating human spirit uses the product of both the male and female gamete—the zygote. The mixture of the content of both nuclei creates a condition of a multi-potential chaos. Out of this state a total unique human being is constituted. Genomes of both nuclei from the parental cells partake in combining spontaneously directed by the spirit-germ. This seed also called the morula potentiates the shape and form for a new human being-Homo Erectus. An incarnating Spirit-being divides into two specific impulses playing a role in embryogenesis. The first split yielding the spirit-germ is "overseer" in the merger of male and female gamete and resulting cell cleavage, morula formation, and finally development of the blastocyst.

With embedding the blastocyst becomes trophoblast nestling within the inner mucosa of the womb. Give or take twenty days the

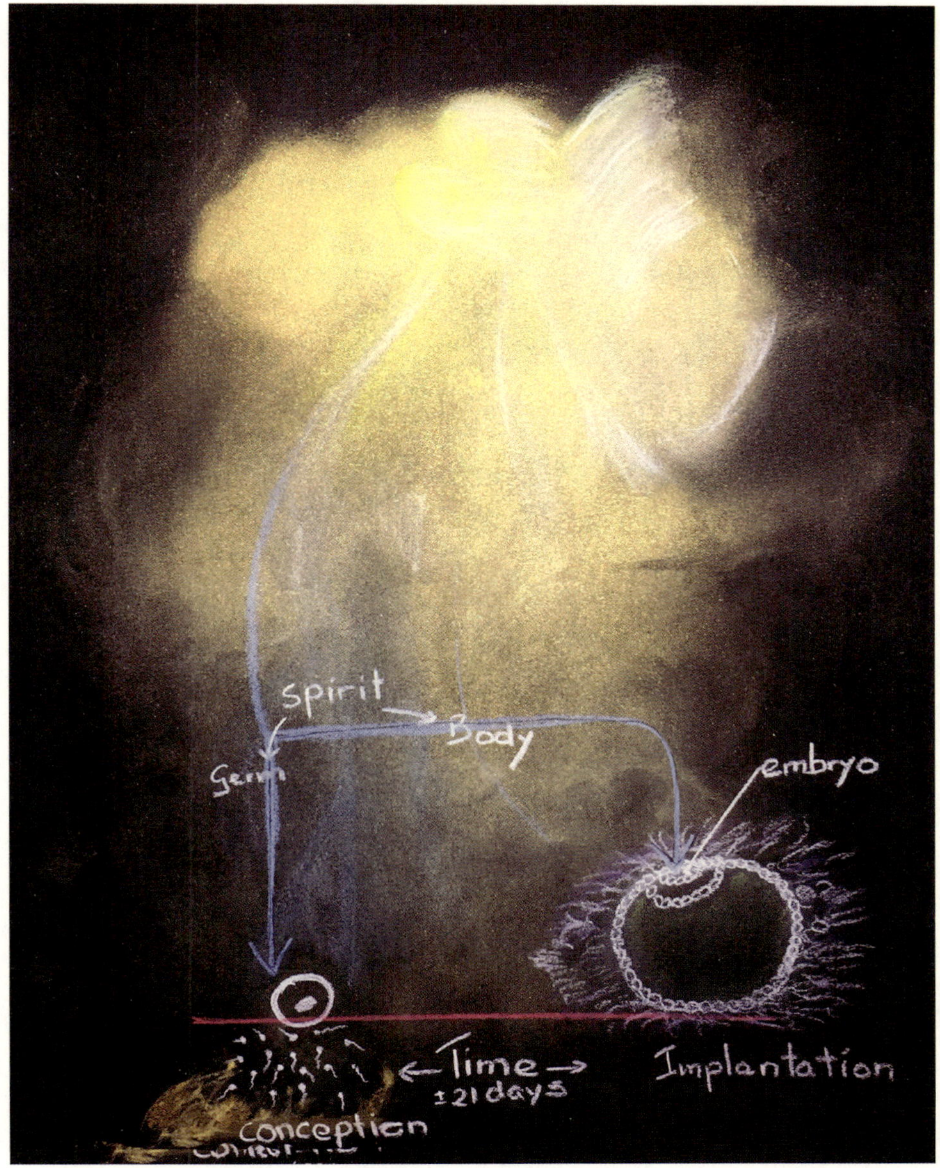

Plate 58: Incarnation of ***The One:*** *two activities and its completion*

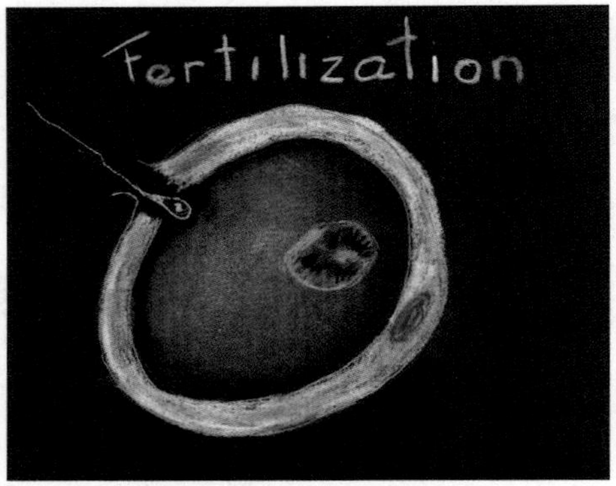

Plate 59: Fertilization

final merger with the Spirit body is completed. Now we observe the formation of a threefold cell structure. From here on specificity and the template of unique characteristics will develop.

Polar opposites are here introduced. The dynamic sounding E(ey) is part instrumental in creating the condition of attraction between opposite gametes. Where the oocyte is exceptionally large, immobile, and filled with cytoplasm, the sperm cell is active, very mobile, and small, carrying only a concentrated nucleus with the twenty-three chromosomes. The gamete donated by the male parent must make a long and arduous journey to its final place of action. The female gamete the oocyte is rich in cytoplasm, and provides an element of form. This pinhead-size egg cell bursts from the ovary during ovulation and is immediately surrounded by the soft tentacle-like protrusions of the fallopian tube (*fimbriae*). This is the place where these two opposite cell structures will meet for conception. The spirit being sojourning in cosmic spaces and for us yet foreign dimensions undergoes a journey from above to below. This movement can also be seen as a crossing over the threshold into a material existence.

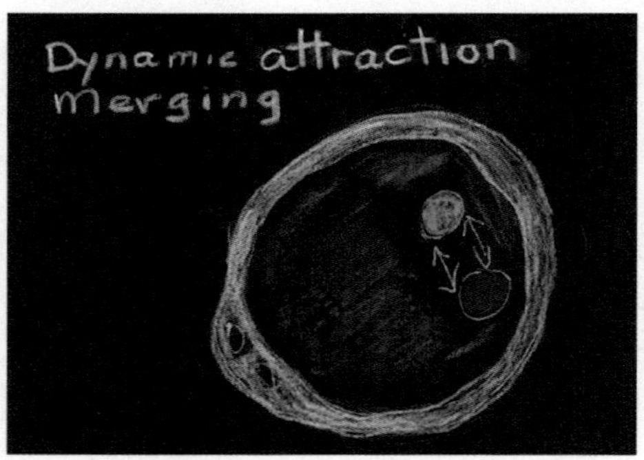

Plate 60: Dynamic attraction

It can be imagined that the mother cell is tucked away in the inner recesses of the female pelvis, an area where negative pressure exists. The perfect round bowl presented as the female pelvic bone structure, in its nature, will spawn a vortex movement whereby the eye becomes a vacuum and asserts a negative pressure or suction on the content. This suction from below enables the sperm to swim deep into the womb, and from above the spirit-being awaiting its merger (incarnation). One can have an imagination that the pelvis becomes like a Grail made ready to receive a substance from beyond the Earth.

We have to realize that the selection of one sperm to penetrate the cell membrane of the oocyte or "mother-cell" is not a haphazard occurrence taking place as a physiological random process (fertilization). Penetration of the female gamete's membrane by the male gamete becomes a spiritual event! The germ cells are joined by the Spirit-germ. Embryogenesis asks for the cooperation of the most important entity in the process of fertilization, the incarnated Spirit-being, the newborn human entity—**The One**. From the second postulate of Hermes Trismegistus we learn:

Postulate II:

> *The below is as the above, the above is as the below to perfect the wonders of **The One**.*

In its successful attempt to reach embodiment in the zygote, **The One** will claim domain of the parental cell. The phases of the first three weeks in the development from a one cell structure to a multi-cell pea-size organism is studied in detail. The

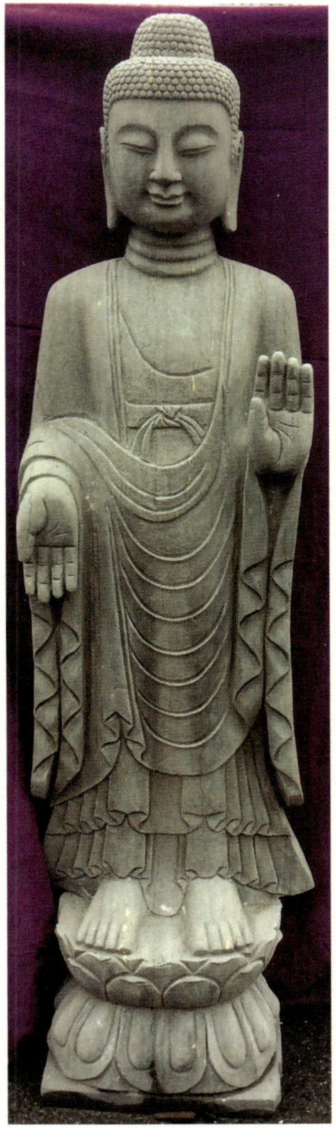

Plate 61: Buddha: above as below

encapsulated nuclear zygote undergoes segmentation cell division to reach a maximum of sixteen cells. This so-called morula can be likened to the plant seed, a cell bundle carrying identical genetic material that is undifferentiated. This cell mass can also be seen as "the wonder of **The One**." These embryonic stem cells can be harvested, processed and donated as material for cloning (differentiated to organ or complete organism).

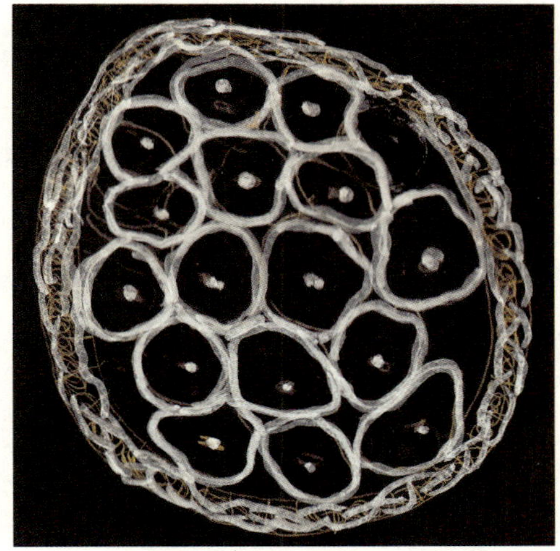

Plate 62: Morula

In a state of metabolic suspension, possessing an **autonomous biological development**, each cell has the capacity to determine the physical development of an identical individual organism. This cluster of sixteen identical cells (morula) is the source for numerous scientific investigations, manipulations and speculations. Not joined by the Spirit Body, it cannot claim individuality. It produces the stem cell, used in regeneration of organ tissue. Cloning makes it possible that identical humanoids can be produced in future laboratories.

In Goethe's *Faust*, the Homunculus embodies the quest for pure spirit to be born into humankind, in sharp contrast to Faust's desire to shed his body and become pure spirit. For Paracelcus (*De Natura Rerum*, 1537), it is a little man who knows everything born from an Alchemical procedure. Goethe's Faust embodies the "little" man with full wisdom of the human being. The Homunculus, in its glass sphere, likened to the morula contains the blueprint for human creation, however not inspirited. Could this allude to the *Philosopher Stone* captivating the imagination of many researchers?

Of interest is the Child Artist's illustration, which places the seed on the left side. In his process of embryogenesis, a distinct humanoid figure is seen in the center. This phase in embryogenesis is where silence reigns, all metabolic activity ceases, the Spirit-germ is suspended. The baton is raised. Creation is watching, holding breath. This is the moment of autonomous biological development.

Once the morula is expelled from the confinement of the tube into the uterine cavity, the germinating power is quickened. Through cyst-making, a distinction arises between the cells that infiltrate and search for nutrients and the cells occupied with embryo-making that divide (Guus van der Bie, *Embryology*). Once the blastocyst becomes part of the uterine wall explosive expansion begins. The

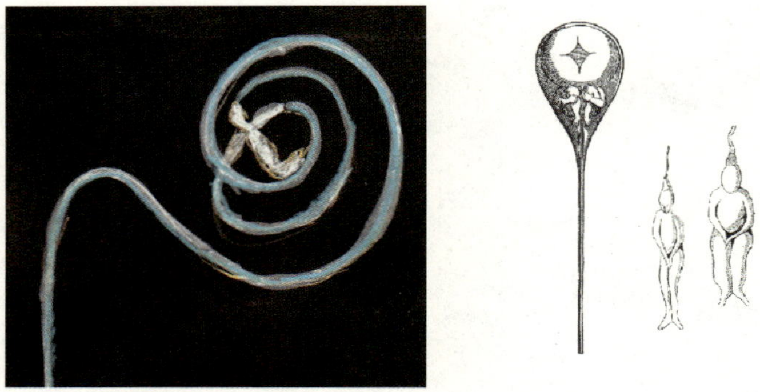

Plate 63: Depictions of the homunculus

embryo (trophocyst) is nineteen days old and the spirit body, hovering over the genesis activity, now joins the development. Incarnation of the Spirit-being **The One** is complete and a new phase in the embryogenesis begins. No doubt the individuation process falls under the vowel sound "I" (ee); however it becomes a vital part of the story that now unfolds.

At the moment the spirit body has joined the expanding developing cell structure, completing the incarnation of **The One,** a germ-disc is recognizable in the inner cell mass. Remarkable is the fact that the cells of these three layers each have a designated function connected to body development. We referred to the threefold constitution of the physical body. In the embryo we see that already in the third week the foundation for this constitution is organized especially where different cell constructions take on responsibility for organ formation. Like the music incites the dancer or the ball activates the game, so through the dynamic activity inherent in growth movements of the three layers ectoderm, mesoderm, and endoderm, the threefold organization in the embryonic organism is established. These layers each will lend an orderly unfoldment with its respective functions in the embryo. The ectoderm, mesoderm, and endoderm layers each contain cells that will execute a specific task. The large orchestra that is made available to **The One** who is the conductor, is of a glorious perfection. The cells of each layer become an instrument that is directed by the forces from "above." In the process of invagination these layers begin to fold, embrace, polarize, and find a designation for their unique role in the development of the embryo. Surrounded by fluid on both sides, the mass now graduates to an embryonic disc and the distinct three layering.

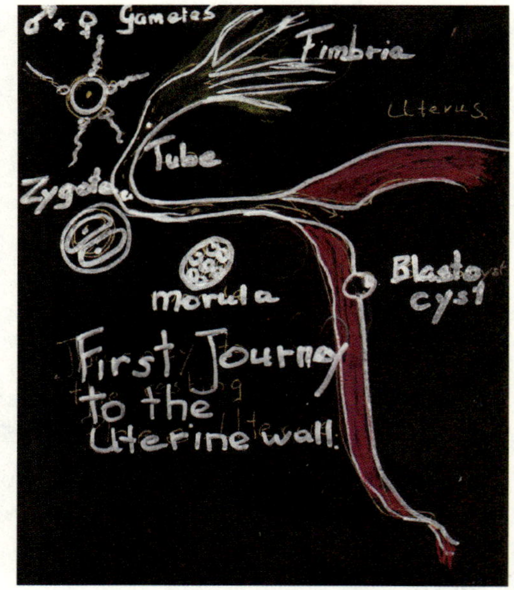

Plate 64: The journey

For instance, the cells of the ectoderm will be responsible for the development of the skin epidermis, the neurons of the central nervous system and pigment cells. The cells of the mesoderm layer are given the task of muscle cell development (heart, uterine, skeletal, and smooth muscle) and red blood cell formation. The endoderm layer contains cells that will be available for the formation of the lung, the liver, the endocrine organs of thyroid and pancreas, and the epithelial cells of all organs. Contemplating the hidden value of threefolding, we meet the evolutionary separation in the soul life-forces of thinking, feeling, and activity of will. Thinking with the "head" assigns the mind as the brain in action. The expression "touching" is often used when an emotion stirs us. Stimulating the sense organ of touch evokes strong feelings. The numerous red blood cells in the skin find their origin in the mesoderm. The cells of the endoderm layer become responsible for excretion, purification, and nutrition.

The One becomes the conductor in the symphony of creating its physical body. The knowing of cosmic wisdom from the vertical in-streaming will govern the execution of the forming process. Music from the heavenly spheres as interpreted through the vowel sounds guide the formation of all the organs step by step.

The creation of the physical body after all becomes an individual task, a mandate from **The One**, with familiarity of this

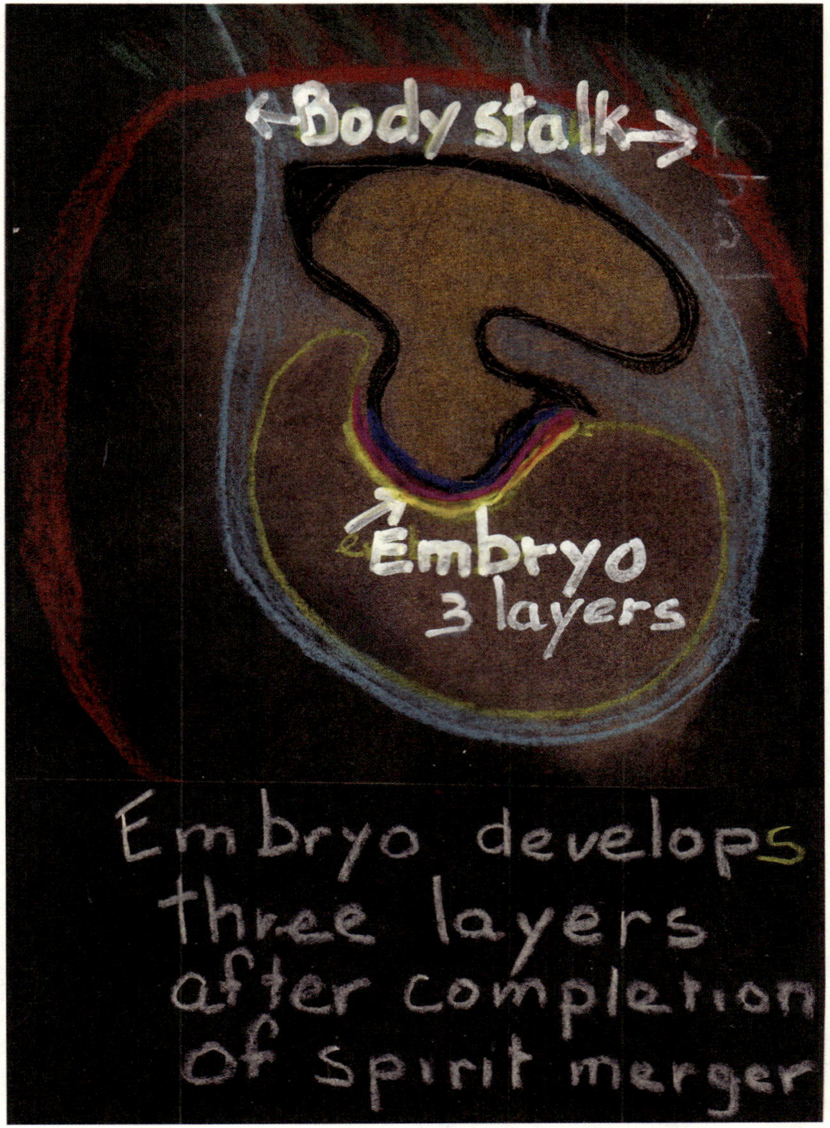

←Body stalk→
Embryo
3 layers
Embryo develops
three layers
after completion
of spirit merger

Plate 65: Body stalk carrying three layers

flowing out of a cosmic knowing as witnessed in the illustrations of the Child Artist. Let us examine the middle section of the template drawing titled embryogenesis. First the helmet of a transparent nature arises from the right side representing symbolically the consolidated mineral earth. This dome with five individual colored hair-like appendages in the front could be interpreted as an artistic presentation of the central nervous system. The five sense organs that first develop belong to the eye, ear, nose, tongue, and skin. The fact that this system functions in a silica reach environment is illustrated by the artist's connection to the Earth's crust, which is composed ninety percent of silicate minerals.

The middle region, drawn in red and orange, occupy a substantial space in the embryonic development. What is obvious is the inter penetration of these two structures in a tentacle-like

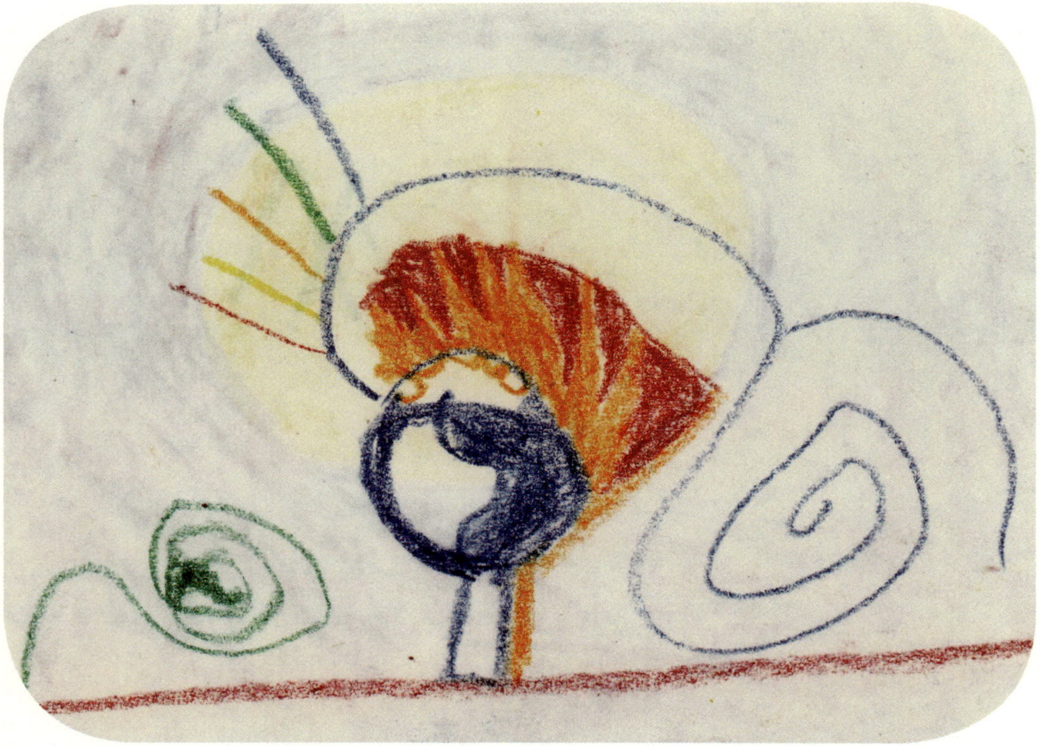

Plate 66: Child Artist's depiction of embryo (fragment)

fashion (formation of somites?). If the dome and red-colored cell mass represent the ectoderm, it is the union between the ectoderm and the mesoderm (orange) that becomes information symbolically represented by the Child Artist. Indeed a process of enclosure of cells from the ectoderm by the mesoderm cells exists. This structure eventually carries the spinal chord embedded in the vertebra.

The artist colors the third layer and its voluminous organ in blue surrounded by a cystic lake. This part of the embryo is firmly connected to the Earth. Five suction cups reach out of the middle mass into a vesicle below. The cells of the endoderm layer take on the function of nutrition, metabolism, and excretion. The heavy mass surrounded by water resembles the liver representing the largest metabolic organ in the embryo. Of all embryonic organs, the liver functions optimum with a very low blood oxygen saturation. The dark-blue color is very well chosen.

Scientifically obtained dissections of numerous human embryos augmented the study of Embryology with accurate information. All students can familiarize themselves with the dynamic process of cell separation and the specific function of cell clusters. The developing embryonic tissue exhibiting sophisticated early displays in the designation of three layers is correlated with the earthly incarnation of the Spirit-body.

Comparison between the drawings of our six-year-old Child Artist and the accurate microscopic information gleaned informs us about a suprasensory process. Unraveling these riddles makes us realize that knowing intricate processes are carried as memories to newborns, assigned to create their own body. After incarnation **The One** becomes the conductor. The baton is raised, in focused expectation, waiting for the moment to lead the orchestra into symphonic music of their own creation. What is brought by the individuality, **The One**, onto the earthly plane? Incarnation as well as reincarnation is an acceptable philosophy. Memories from the past are brought by **The One** and stored in the etheric body, the body fluids with which the embryo is surrounded. Spiritual content is stored during the time of development in utero. The young Child Artist brings us the hidden memories of learnings beyond adult understanding.

Postula III:

> *And as all things come from* ***The One*** *from the meditation of* ***The One*** *, So all things are born from* ***The One****, by adaptation.*

Full authority is given to **The One** in the third postulate of the Emerald Tablet. Here Hermes Trismegistus inaugurates the process of **The One** completing its incarnation. Full power is bestowed to **The One** who can oversee the development of its own body. Only after the chaos created in the first process of chromosomal blending has been attained, authenticity is established. Order out of Chaos in the parental nucleus means adaptation.

What is the relationship to the Mother at this stage of development? The embryo occupies space not larger than one to two centimeters, has its own genetic signature foreign to the host and no exchange of blood is found. The nutrition of the embryo is secured by the nutrient osmosis in the cell vacuities present in the uterine wall. The embryo is a parasite, however not rejected but embraced by the mother. Could it be that the integration of the human being with its fourfold activity of warmth, light, living water with chemical exchange procures a foundation for acceptance by the mother? The blissful nature of the expecting mother is not surprising. New life is a gift. Let us proceed to the fourth Postula.

Postula IV:

> *Its father is the Sun, its mother Is the Moon; the Wind carries it in its belly, its nurse is the Earth.*

With this postulate Hermes Trismegistus introduces us to the four Aristotelian elements, fire, air, water, and earth, which deserve attention regarding the constitution of **The One**. The four-body concept was first discussed as a foundation stone in Anthroposophy. The sources of the four elements used for contemplating the fourth postulate of the Emerald Tablet are rich and meaningful. Keep in mind that the total postulate was given to the students of Alchemy involved with their own purification and spiritual growth. Repetitive study of the content would change the soul-life into a desired state of openness and understanding.

The cadaver is a presentation of only the mineral chemistry referred to as dust or salt of the earth. Functioning as a living entity requires animation derived from the infusion of living water, the circulation of air and the penetration of fire providing warmth. Life is donated to **The One** by the parental gametes of opposing forces. The physiognomy of the male gamete is small and mobile as if stirred by centrifugal forces of the radiating warmth and air. The female gamete moves sluggishly, and the cell is filled with living water in which the chemical exchanges dominate. **The One** penetrates the gametes to acquire substance (earth as nurse) and with three other aspects enables completion of the fourfold etheric body. Father Sun donating the aspect of warmth/fire and Mother Moon donating living water and Wind as carrier of the air in the belly.

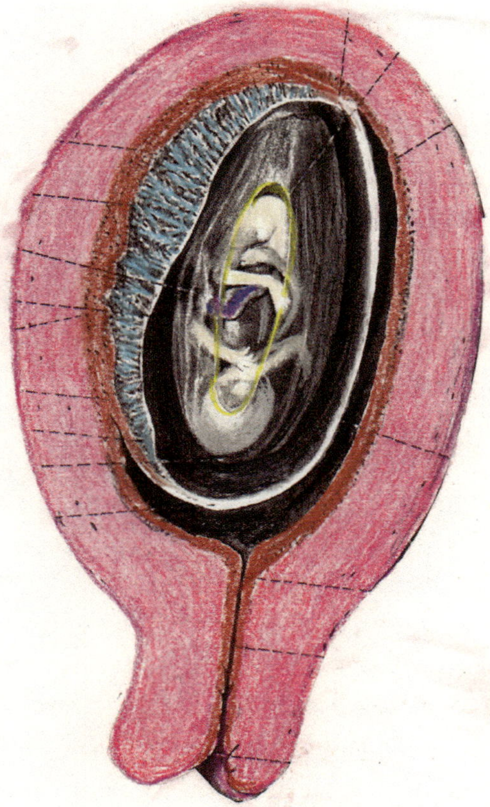

Plate 67: Embryonic developed fetus tucked in womb

Throughout the first weeks of pregnancy **The One's** contortions can be compared to a balloon dancing in the air. Opposing currents give rise to a three dimensional dynamics that ultimately ends with the well-known tucked in, flexed, fetal presentation at the end of three months.

The image of the embryonal urge for cell growth, differentiation into zones, division into distinct functions, responsive placement into opposite poles that cannot unfold orderly unless pressure from the outside continues, places the observer in the middle of a moving marvel of wonders. A memory of the sequences in these movements will contribute to an enrichment of our own imaginative powers, which is so necessary for the future.

It stands to reason that the new incarnation (spiritualized primitive embryonic body), can assert a birds-eye view and uses the directing forces streaming in from cosmic spaces as music from the spheres, with the suprasensory organs still available. Examples of these forces were already demonstrated in the Chladny figures (1835). I want to introduce the body of work by a well-known physician and student of Anthroposophy, Hans Jenny (Cymatics). The experiments to demonstrate the effect of sound vibration on solid substances, were painstakingly photographed for posterity. This body of work can be seen as groundbreaking in the illustration of formative forces. His insight into the problems of modern physiology and biology spurred the experimental field to include the effects of vibrations in concrete medium. This experimental phenomenology is named *Cymatics*.

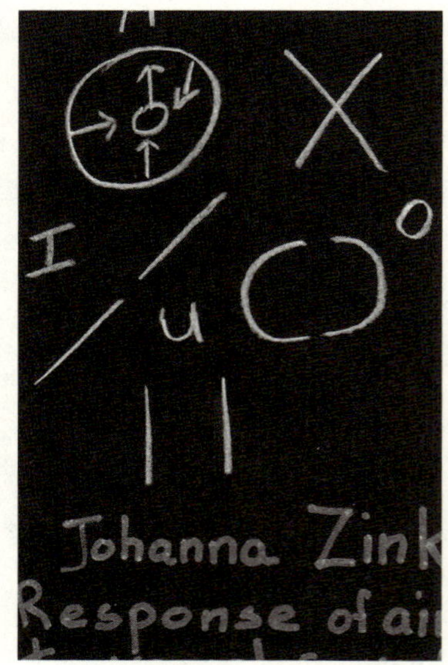

Plate 68: Vowels in air

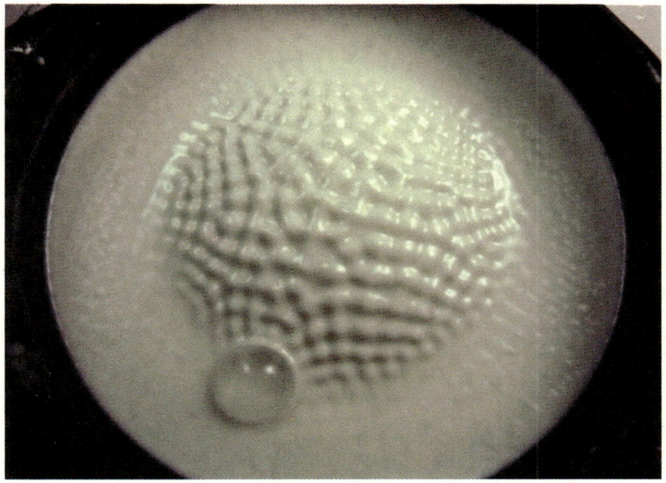

Plate 69: Cymatics in fluid

Johanna Zinke, a student of Rudolf Steiner also conducted independent research using smoke to develop creative vowel patterns from speech. Her work enforces the creative shaping of matter through tonal resonance in the head of the human being.

These illustrations are examples of the potential that vibrations induce on a medium. The shape, density, size, form, all are dependent on the material being excited, its shape and form, as well as the highlighting material (sand, smoke, dye), and the sound frequency to which it is exposed. The spiritualized primitive embryonic body (The One) finds itself in a self-regulating domain.

Embryogenesis is experienced as a journey through the ***kingdoms of the Earth***. The male and female gamete just before their demise, meaning if fusion would not take place, are doomed to death. This fact introduces us to the mineral world. Being on the verge of not being enlivened is a near death experience. After this we witness a seed existence, the morula, which is then followed by the image of rapid growth we witness for instance in a mushroom, all images of the plant world. The process of invagination to form gastrula or a pocket belongs to the development as a member in the animal kingdom.

The body of the embryo is animalized as soon as the spirit germ and spirit body merge as one, to become whole as the spiritual entity in the embryo of **The One**.

In natural science, Ontogeny describes the history of the development of an individual. In the animal kingdom it pertains to the developmental history of an organism within its own lifetime, as distinct from phylogeny, which refers to the evolutionary history of the species. Darwinism underscores ontogeny, human-species evolving on the rungs of the ladder of the animal kingdom by adaptation. However the argument that the phases in phylogeny have ceased, once the human species entered evolution, has validity. Suddenly all the species of the animal kingdom can be seen as stepping stones toward the ultimate goal of the Earth becoming the habitat for humanity (Homo Erectus). In the phylogeny of the human embryo we find phases where the biological stages are reenacted such as plant seed, the fungoid imitation, the early amphibian life, and zoological representations toward the higher mammals, ending very early in the embryogenetic process when the distinct features for the upright man declares itself. The gestalt of uprightness distinguishes the human from the ape-man. The volume of cranial content enables the human to connect with an all-encompassing wisdom of which in the present little is understood. But it is the heart that will become

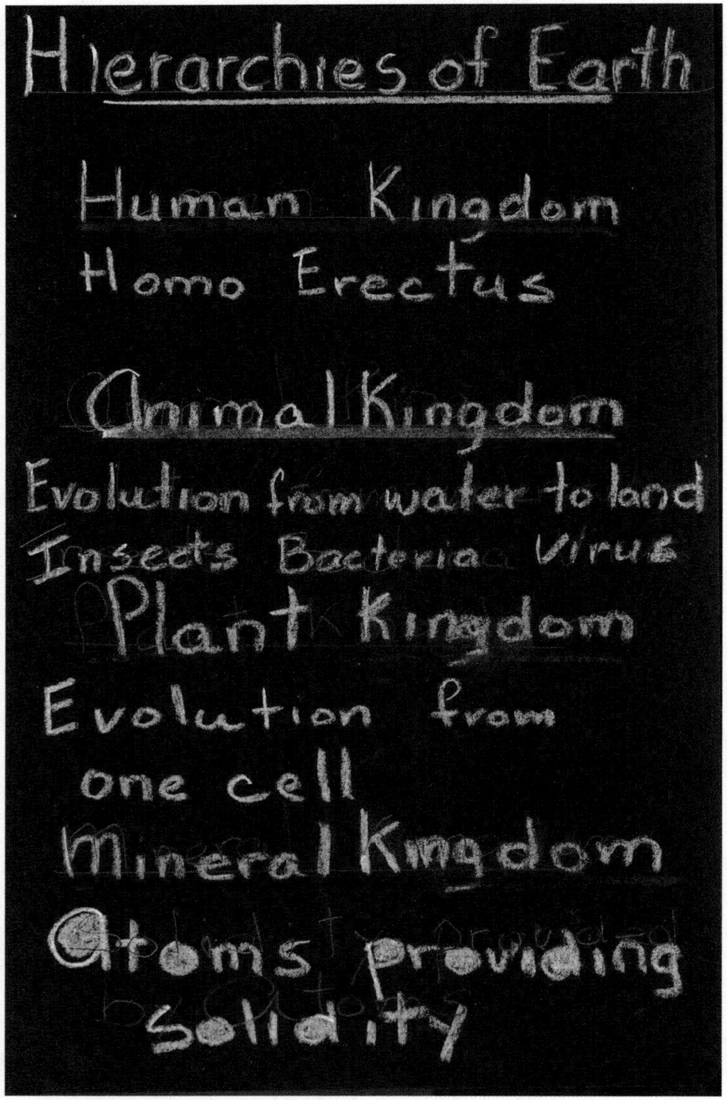

Plate 70: Hierarchies of Earth

the center of all human efforts. This challenging statement becomes a new imagination, underwriting a thinking in the vertical dimension. Surely the Child Artist has made us aware of the wonders in the heart with his drawing (ref. plate 3).

It is recognized that the fetal tissue remains surrounded and continues to produces an environment containing exceptionally high silicon content. One wonders about the reason for such an aberrance, unless it is used by **The One** to strengthen the senses (hear the Music of the Spheres). One can imagine that the high silicon content of the tissue enhances the transmission of suprasensory messages from outer space. The embryonic tissue becomes an antenna.

Awed by the rapid turn of events in the first few weeks of the embryonic development, Hermes Trismegistus describes the process in his fifth postulate:

Postulate V:

> *It is the Father of all wonders of the whole world, Its power is perfect, when it is transformed into Earth.*

The role of father in a culture of three thousand years ago (when the postulate appeared) was bestowed on a protective leader, usually a person or deity who was supreme (half God, half human) worthy in the role of a God who had a full understanding of the life processes in the world it inhabited, performed miracles, and received adoration from this world. In this postulate "It" is assigned the role of "Father." **The One** is named as the originator of the wonders he himself performs in the process of incarnation. The adoring exclamation over this postulate, praising the power of perfection in the task of incarnating, is not lost on the reader. Adoration is deserved because the wonders performed in the process of transformation from The Spirit incarnation into the human body are sublime.

Could Embryogenesis as performed by **The One** be praised because it announces a new step in the evolution of the Earth and the human? Praised is not only "its" ability to incarnate, but the explicit potential of **The One** to create a human body in its perfection as the culmination in Creation. Connecting the "whole world" with the appearance of the human on Earth could give Genesis as written by Moses an unexpected twist. The Sophia, present in the human soul created the sphere of the Earth for the human being to inhabit a physical solid body. Spiritual Science assigns to the Earth three previous existences that of Old Saturn, Old Sun, Old Moon, and finally the Earth (Occult Science Rudolf Steiner). Each of these conditions led to the intensification of solid states. What was once warmth became light through air, then life in water, and in the final stage, a hardened mineral solid mass, the world of molecules and chemistry on the Earth. Humanity is a witness to this creative process and incorporates it in embryogenesis.

This postulate confirms the recognition of power given to human beings as the center of creation. The two conscious individualities participating in this marvel and giving witness thereof do have an understanding of Genesis and Embryo Genesis. Humanity recognizes these beings in the names of Moses and Hermes Trismegistus. The final destination for humanity is not a return to the heavens but a transformed Earth. The assignment is clear. Only collective humanity can and will transform the Earth. How? The remainder of the postulates will give clear insight into future expectations.

At the moment of birth the fetus emerges out of the water and becomes a land dweller, with the necessity to breath in the atmospheric air. The lung used for the first time after the birth, can be assigned as the organ for living on the Earth, the final step in the incarnating process of the individuality. Deployment of the alveolar pockets is an indication that the fetus has become an Earth citizen. As Goethe states "The Eye is made by the light for the light." So can we also reason that the breathing organ is made for inspiration by the spirit—**The One** (IN-SPIRE). The One becomes

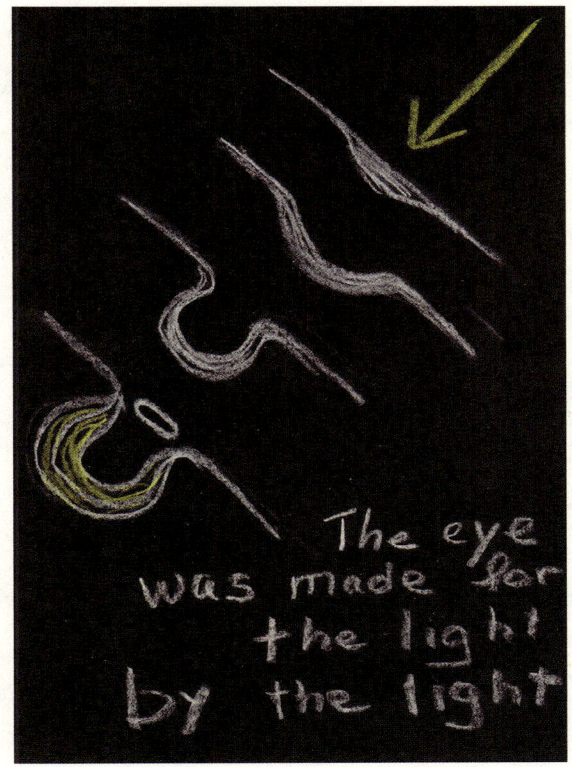
The eye
was made for
the light
by the light

Plate 71: Process of invagination

a citizen of the Earth by dent of partaking in the inhalation of the first gift of Earth, it's atmosphere. Spirit becomes independently human with the first inspiration. At the other side of birth, the opposite process, the last breath, at death, expiration, inaugurates a process of excarnation from the realm of Earth and a birth or stepping over into cosmic dimensions.

The Birthing of the Child

In the last forty years of practicing medicine in Columbia County, New York, the most exciting challenge certainly was the accompaniment of the pregnant mother and assisting her in the event of parturition. Usually it was the home birth desired by the parents, and as a practitioner of anthroposophic medicine in a rural area, I always felt it was an honor to participate in a true learning process. Being a mother myself and giving birth in the mid-1960s in a sterile, cold hospital environment, I certainly had sympathies for the courageous woman who wanted to make a conscious choice to change the reception of the new earthling into an environment of warmth and joy.

In my personal history I remember the battle to secure a natural birth and the right to breast-feed in a calculating medical system in the beginning of my path to motherhood. Even as a medical professional it ended up that I was shunned or rather left to my own devices for all pre- and postpartum care, a bit of a nightmare. But then I did have the strong memory of my parents who, both as physicians, had delivered women in their homes, in the late thirties and throughout the German occupation in northern Holland, which was not an easy time. Out of the hundreds of deliveries they assisted there were no incidents reported of loss of life for the mother or other complications caused by neglect. From them I sensed an all-pervading strength and levelheadedness and the capability of allowing natural events for the mother to unfold. They had learned about patience, especially, patience for the uterus to do its work, recognizing this muscle as an integral part of the birthing process. Anatomically the wall of the uterus has a dominant layer of smooth muscle fibers, both longitudinal and circular, which undergo a hypertrophy as well as an increase in the number of fibers up to twenty-four times during the ten lunar months of pregnancy.

The female hormone estrogen stimulates the smooth muscle fibers to undergo hypertrophy and hyperplasia. The muscle fiber is unique in its response to hormonal messages. Contraction of the muscle can be stimulated by the hormone oxytocin, a pituitary gland extraction, and prostaglandins. This occurs naturally when the fetus' birth time has arrived and he/she is assigned the role as the captain of the ship named "natural childbirth." Contraction of these muscles allows expulsion of the content to take place not only through shortening of the body of muscles, but also by stretching the tight mouth or cervix so that the fetus can move down the birth canal and be vaginally delivered. The growth of the fetus cannot be separated from the astounding development of the muscular mass of the uterine organ, which is not only the incubator for the fetus for ten lunar months, but will also become the tool of expulsion for the child in the birthing process. It is established that the tools for the child-controlled delivery are available in the form of hormonal secretion by the mother, oxytocin, or the prostaglandins excreted by the fetal membranes.

The understanding that each delivery is different and unique has an absolute validity if we take into consideration that each birthing human being **The One** is a unique entity breathing the air of the Earth. For those of us who have assisted in births, this diverse experience is not a surprise. We experience that the spontaneous relaxed birth becomes the expression of the being we assist in our midst.

How often did mothers remark that there was a correlation between the child's first introduction to life on Earth (expression through birthing) and the signature of the new being in the making of footprints on the Earth.

We notice the correlation between the progression of the natural birth and the nature and needs of **The One**. For instance, in those children who know their wants, who are direct in their communications and are quickly satisfied, a delivery that was strong and short with no nonsense was experienced. Juxtaposed we have a birthing process that naturally unfolded slower, as if the child needed to take its time, an introduction for the parents to the real signature of this new being. A mother can experience both variations of the process at different births, indicating that the child must be heard during the process of birthing. Here the mother is given an opportunity to acquaint herself with the character or soul configuration of this child. In the child's activity of dominating the uterine muscle contraction, the will forces, decisiveness, and eventual enthusiasm for life are demonstrated.

Foremost, the work of the birth assistant becomes twofold. First one learns that the natural childbirth can be divided into stages connected with the movement of the fetus into the birth canal. The completion of the first stage sets the second stage in motion, and so on. The assistant works with the parameters of time and progress set out through knowledge and experience. If it is accepted and understood that the child sets the pace, the assistant has two masters to serve: the Child and the Mother.

It is the mother that has to be convinced during the delivery, that a part of her body does not belong to her. She needs to donate it to the incoming being so that the process of expulsion can be enhanced. In this letting go, an enormous act of trust is established. Can I, as the woman in parturition, accept that the individual being, in the act of birthing, does not want to cause me pain? Does a natural process for cooperation exist? Yes!

As the uterine contractions become longer and more intense, a twilight zone can be entered into, a consciousness where in the mother is able to concentrate on the prolongation of the individual contractions, a relaxed trusting, an unconditional state of donating, standing back to allow the child to take over. In assisting we need to be present for the mother and father in a process of an unending sacrificial act.

An image that may be helpful is the word play between *Hystera* and Hysteria. Both are Greek words, the root *Hystera* means Uterus. *Hyster-i-a* is a mental manifestation in which a second personality of emotional instability takes over. *Hysteria* could be the state of losing it during parturition, the process of birth. Of course, hysteria is not only for the parents but also for the obstetric team. That is the time when modern intervention is being proposed. With the promise and belief that the modern medical system truly heals and does no harm, we as consumers trade in our rights and ability to self heal, along with the choice for dignified alternatives. There is no doubt in my mind that medical intervention may be justified even for obstetrical care. Witnessing, the astounding rise of surgical intervention, promising the mother a pain-free, speedy, programmed delivery, the time has come for women to go back to the drawing board and reconnect with what childbirth is all about.

I have attempted to provide a new image from my own experience—an image that recognizes the triumph of natural childbirth for both the adult and the new Earth being. **The One** can find the intimacy and ecstasy of an experience that inspires the initiation of a parental unit. In the preparation for this portentous event we can use the following meditation throughout the pregnancy.

I stand before you
New miracle of life
You entered my being
And I await in awe
Your first footprint
In this your new life.

"Our children come through us; they are not of us"
—**Kahlil Gibran**, *The Prophet*

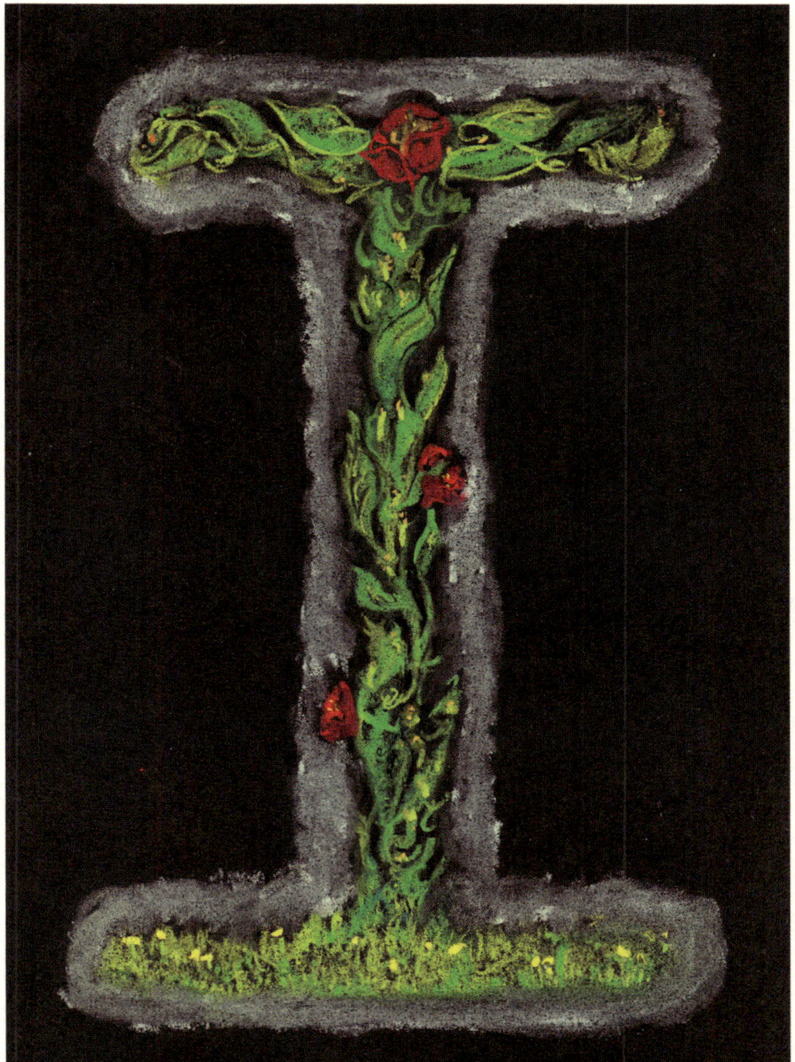
Plate 72: Sound I as depiction

Sound I

The *I* as a vowel is easily identified as a gesture in which light streams down from the cosmos into the human being through an outstretched right arm, bathing and surrounding the human figure with a projection of independence and identity. An imagination of forces streaming out from Earth, penetrating the feet, legs and pelvis, straightening the posture in the upright position, is also familiar.

In the previous sections, illustrations and explanations were provided in which the incarnating process of **The One** was introduced. The historic reality of Alchemy and the collective memory thereof, the recognition of a creative process from the "Above" to the "Below" whether in the soul-spirit or physical embryogenesis becomes source material during our contemplation in the "silent" time. Throughout the whole of creation the music of the spheres sounding as the vibrational vowel sounds accompany the steps.

Birthing provides joy and promise of possibilities. Contemplation of Death provokes uncertainties and fear. One cannot help but recognize that evolution is the journey of THE ONE throughout dimensions, a sojourn toward an ultimate goal. One even may be able to grasp the ultimate outcome in this glorious event; however, most of the time one gets stuck on a plane of time and space being subjected to the mundane and personal crisis, "the whale of tears," experienced on a daily basis.

This section is centered on "I" fulfilling its task while breathing the air of Earth. The burden of the cloak of personality, the lack of insight into one's own imperfections, the frustration to discover that with years of outward gain, inner changes for a spirit knowledge has

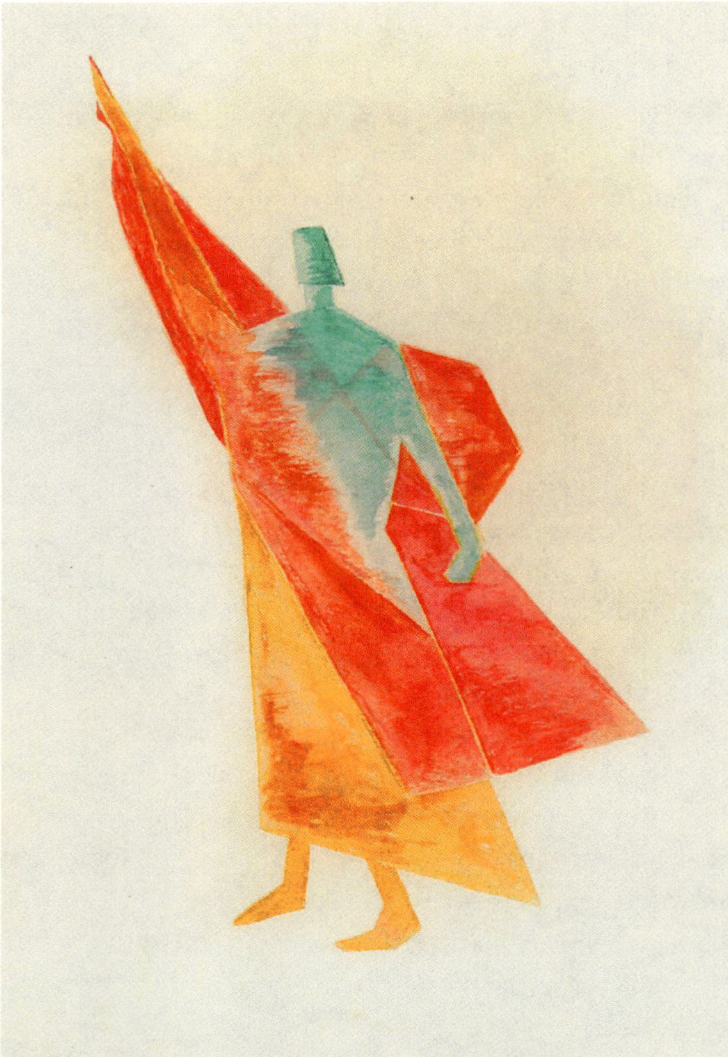

Plate 73: Eurythmy gesture of I

mostly been eluded, all of this must be examined while in the vibrational section of *"I."*

In my own biography the role as a physician placed me in a position of trust and intimacy. In the role as obstetrician, the intimate birthing process was accompanied for at least one hundred deliveries. Many a youth meets me now after twenty-five years knowing that I was present during their first breath of life. This creates a mood of trust, a sense of continuity and availability in a field beleaguered by institutions. What is more intimate than the visit where the patient is facing his/her own aging and dying process? I do not turn away from extending myself, sharing with the patient an imagination of a birthing process in altered dimensions, a reality wherein a transformation instead of cessation can be enlivened by an image of a new birth.

The dying patient on chemotherapy pleads for help; it becomes impossible for him or her to control the natural death process. He or she cannot consciously embrace the process of excarnation. They become a witness to failure of severing the bond between the physical body and the life body. That is precisely the goal of pharmaceutical intervention, to strengthen the attachment between these two bodies so that a longer life is guaranteed. The quality of life is not questioned. As the "I" of humanity grows stronger, questions of immortality will emerge and need to be addressed not only by the spiritual guide, but the health care worker who is in charge of any hospice situation.

The patient's biography is examined as the stepping-stones **The One** encountered from cradle to grave. I also frequently use the autobiographical stories experienced throughout my life to illustrate the objective lawfulness of the Science of the Spirit also in my life.

The reality of space is a conscious experience for me. Through my eye I can see the light. Through my ear I can hear variations of tone. I can touch the solid objects and feel the quality of surfaces. My senses are the instruments used in soul awakening during social intercourse on the horizontal plane. Total silence in the outside world, would equate to a cessation of all stimuli on the senses of the body. Overstimulation of one or two sense organs can cause distraction and prevents the growing child to discover its inherent human potential in privacy without outer interference. The small child is unable to move and control its surrounding and is literally at the mercy of the sensitivity of its parents. Inner silence in adults is practiced during prayer or meditation.

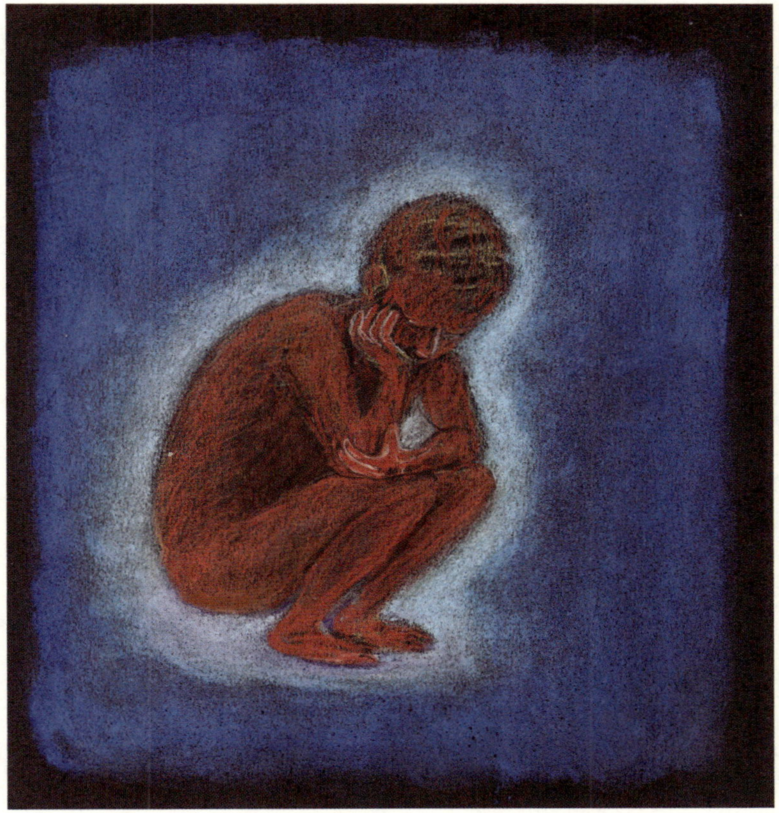

Plate 74: Discover soul activity

Biographically I was blessed with less distraction then usual since both parents were professionals and as a policy left the baby mostly alone. A childcare nurse was our daily companion. I have no memory of my little sister; I do have visions of being sickly and having a cot next to my mother's bed. When awake it was noticed that there was alertness to my surroundings, even a curiosity for the activity around me. In an objective interpretation ever since birth, at the moment of one's first breath one can claim becoming an earthling, with the capacity to use the senses, making percepts, gathering and storing memories. To think my own thoughts and fashion concepts unadulterated by influences from the outer world was and still is my prerogative as **The One**. Silence in which percepts and memories can be re-evaluated is essential for the growing child in order to develop and recognize a sense for truth, beauty, and goodness. These are not inborn human qualities but are acquired in the experience of a state of independence separate from the parental, hovering, doting, and often emotionally needy adult. Through the fleeting pain, fear, and threats, suffering is indeed experienced but resolved with the certainty of a reunion and always a safe home and parental succor.

Is it a requirement to be exposed to the pain of separation? In the silence of the suffering, many aspects of soul responses are developed and digested to become the tapestry of a rich emotional life. The child can learn that there is a difference between what is on the outside and what is within itself. It meets in its day consciousness a duality. One role is the part of its being acting out with a desire to be noticed, with an assigned placement in a family, pleasing and socializing. In other words a child who learns the boundaries and limitations set up by the outside world also becomes aware that there are thoughts and feelings within itself. Thoughts not shared with the outside world, private thoughts. What one thinks and feels will become a part of one's unique biography. The word adulterated is so appropriate here because it is the adult that interferes with the pure expression of the child. Many grownups become unsettled when sitting still. They are prone to ignore the necessity of quiet time for introspection. It is in this fear they hope to protect the children from the same fate. Little does such a parent realize that the solution lies with the child's rich inner life, an emotional state learned through the gift of independence and respected boundaries for both parties concerned. It must be recognized we must protect children (**The Ones**) from undue interference by adults. Their right to privacy is unassailable. Only in such an atmosphere the truth of a vertical reality can break through from higher spheres. What is an example of these truths?

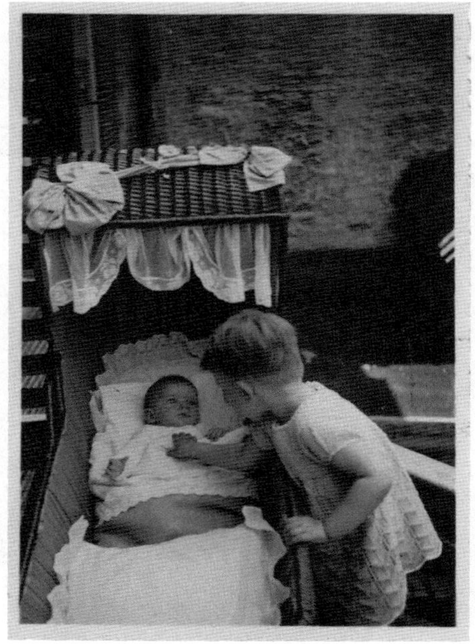

Plate 75: Two sisters

This brings me to a story of a little girl who was overjoyed with the baby sister had just delivered. She requested to her parents that she be left alone with the newborn. Questioning why, she answered "Before she forgets, she will tell me the stories she brought down from heaven." I am reminded here that children are young human beings. Their soul processes of thinking, feeling, and acting are not developed to full maturity. This evokes the impatience of many a parent; however, no parent can assume that to be grown up makes one better. Children understand each other and the bond between them is stronger then we as adults can ever imagine.

At the age of five, as a little girl, I was graced with a suprasensory clairaudient meeting. Far from this changing my life, I had the consciousness not only to experience the voice making a clear statement: "I WAS — I AM — I WILL FOREVER BE," but to question the voice as follows. *Anneke* (my childhood Dutch name), *do not forget this encounter. Here I stand. I am now five years old.* And while looking down on my little frame: *What am I going to do in this small female body?* An overwhelming burden is such a meeting where something larger makes one recognize the insignificance of the horizontal existence. Then the incidence passes into the deep recesses of the child soul but it is never forgotten. It remains a biographical building block on which my whole life's philosophy is resting and later can unfold. When I ask my father at the age of eight if there is a likelihood that we visit the Earth more then once, he immediately refers me to the Indian religious texts where spirit is accepted as an eternal entity and reincarnation is acceptable.

The choice of parent was "right on," is it not so? I as **The One** was protected but remained free from all indoctrinations during my growing years. Only at the age of twenty-one I had a curiosity to study Theosophy but was not a joiner. So what really happened during this timeless experience? It was as if a part of me, I designated as a higher, wiser being, wanted to remind me of the insignificance of mortality. Later I learned through the temple mysteries known in Spiritual Science about the meeting required from pupils during their initiation into Egyptian temples. The teacher, named here the Hierophant of the Temple would guide the pupil in a deep sleep, close to a death experienced for three days. Once moving in the astral world of the dead, the pupil meets The Sphinx, a crouching composite animal with a human head, a lion-like body, limbs and hoofs of a bull, its body covered with wings. Meeting the sphinx is an occult experience described as a path of initiation in the Egyptian temples at least three thousand years in the past. Again it was the Hierophant as teacher and leader of the spiritual school that guided pupils in their final quest toward spiritual initiation that afforded them deeper knowing of the "SELF." The pupils would subject themselves to a temple sleep lasting three days. Extensive training in physical hygiene, emotional restraint, and the understanding of the nether worlds (death) were all requirements that ultimately led up to this final journey, a journey dedicated to the departed souls and an introduction to immortality. This being remained heavily veiled but revealed itself to pupils with a stern voice and the same declaration I was able to hear: *"I was—I am—I will forever be —No one shall lift my veil!"*

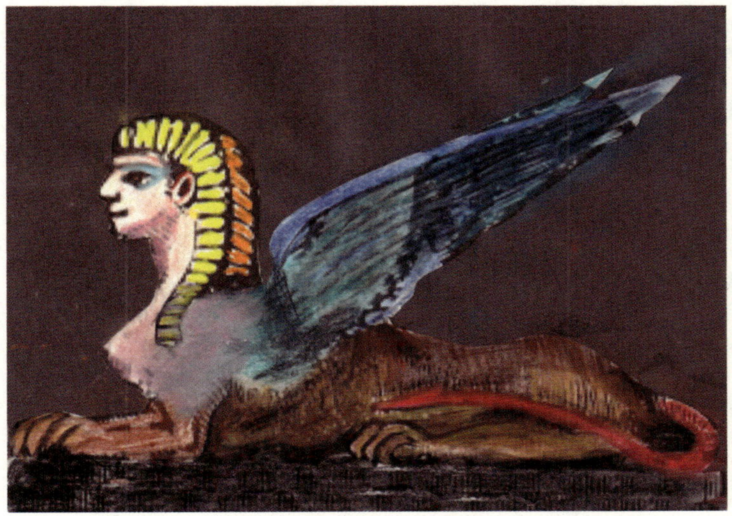

Plate 76: Sphinx

The last phrase however was a warning. What could the veil of secrecy be? Remember that these stringent rituals were performed more than two thousand years ago. The outcome was not always positive, for some postulates did not return from the visit to the nether world. Their sojourn during the temple sleep (astral world) could not be completed and they had to leave this world to reincarnate at a later date. That was exactly the secret of the veil! In those times any investigation into previous incarnations was strictly forbidden. So there is an evolutionary change in the spirit awakening. The opera by Amadeus Mozart, *The Magic Flute,* gives us a very accurate reenactment of this journey. It was the sphinx who carried the secret of past and future lives behind the veil, the veil of forgetfulness. Today, can we lift that veil through our own volition and inner work? How much has changed for the human beings born today in the Western civilization. Kali Yuga, the Iron Age, ended in the late eighteen hundreds. The veil of secrecy was lifted. Gone are the days of backroom séances, secret teachings from the East, and even the spiritual consultant who pretends to know other person's previous lives. Independence in one's own spiritual journey is vouchsafed.

Immortality is a fact! This idea is difficult for people to accept. An atheist living in the materialistic world has physical limitation including the reality of death combined with the fact that no after-life exists. It becomes the knowing that will give us certainty of life after death. Believing (religion) will not suffice for an inquisitive mind; belief does not provide a certainty. To believe is a personally subjective sentiment that has no place in study, exploration, and investigation of the human potential and Truth. Do the knowers have to convince the believers or vice versa? That exactly is a burning question for me and perhaps for all of the persons who were able to enter the higher worlds and had glimpses of truths that could give meaning to earthly existence (ref. plate 29).

Do I have to convince the other person of a reality of which they are not aware? Do I wait until they invite me into their intimate inner explorations? When will a reversal in spiritual attitude manifest in the Western civilizations? Are the natural sciences as taught in our academic establishments the biggest distractors for the young generations? The young also have to deal with a virtual reality the computer has to offer. Will there eventually be a curriculum created for these pupils that would introduce them to Spiritual Science? This will only happen when the student asks for this. I remain open-minded to all changes that can occur.

Experience with our Child Artist has given much support and an example for the future. His individuality is present in all his illustrations. He tells us of pre-earthly travels from far expanses, relationships with planetary hosts, and about his friend the "guardian angel." He has given evidence of lives in the past at which time he experienced research as an alchemist, and shows remarkable knowledge of human genesis. No other person could present us with what he gave in this stage of his life. The personality still needed to unfold for which a span of another two times seven years is needed. Only at the end of his twentieth year the individual would feel the urge to incarnate in the prepared vessel.

Seven-year Phases in Child Maturation

There is a logical interpretation of the biographical years used by the spiritual scientists (ref. plate 13). When used it brings order in labeling the years of human development. It is known that the body cells have a seven-year renewal cycle. Blood cells live much more briefly and take no part in this discussion. If we can take this seven-year period as a ground rule we could also imagine that we have received a new body at seven, (change of teeth), at fourteen (development of sexual organs), and at twenty-one (social maturity). Being aware of the cosmic imprint on all of humanity, the planetary spheres of Moon, Mercury, Venus, Sun, Mars, Jupiter, and Saturn are reflected in this analysis. Understand that the

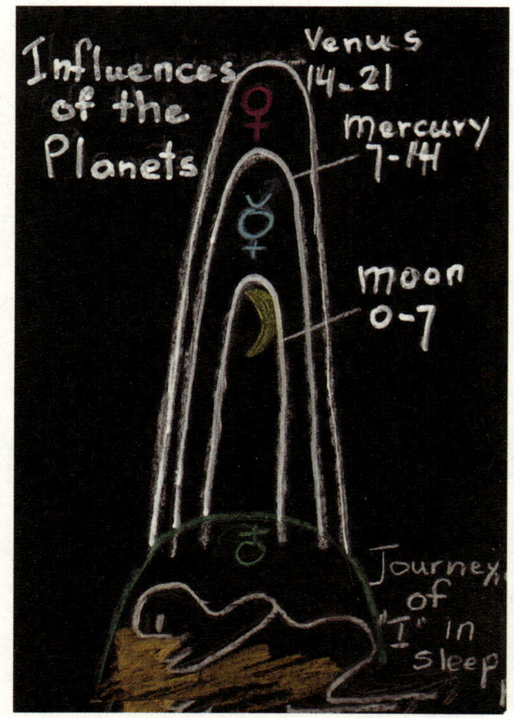

Plate 77: Journey of "I" in sleep (0–21 years)

physical bodies of these planets play no role, but the guidance and cosmic influences from these spheres are taken very serious.

With a living imagination the Moon is identified as a reflector. Not only does it reflect information from Earth but also becomes the reflecting power for the whole universe. The metal connected with this body is silver. The brain is the organ of reflection in the physical body. As this function predominates in the first seven years we can deduce that it brings knowledge out of cosmic spaces into the glue substance in the first seven years of child development. In sleep its attention is focused on the Moon. Every moment the child loses itself in this sphere it receives instruction on how to build the physical body, strengthening memories and renewing connections with cosmic hosts. This intimate relationship ends with the falling out of the milk teeth. The Moon period functions as body builder.

It is through the Tooth Fairy the child is introduced to an higher sphere, the sphere of Mercury. The development in the next seven years stands very much in the sign of Mercury, not the physical planet but a world of mercury forces overseeing humanity from a higher dimension (cosmic spaces). These cosmic beings as a part of the Hierarchies are recognizable in their gifts of good health, playfulness, and laughter, inducing a mercurial disposition in the child often bordering on banality. A sanguine nature sometimes inducing stealing but must not be interpreted as a moral defect in the child, rather as an imitation of the god Mercury, the deity blessing traders, money-lenders, and thieves. Of course the metal mercury influences the life function in the physical body. We could introduce here the etheric body as the recognizable sheath beyond the physical that is in need of attention in the developing human being.

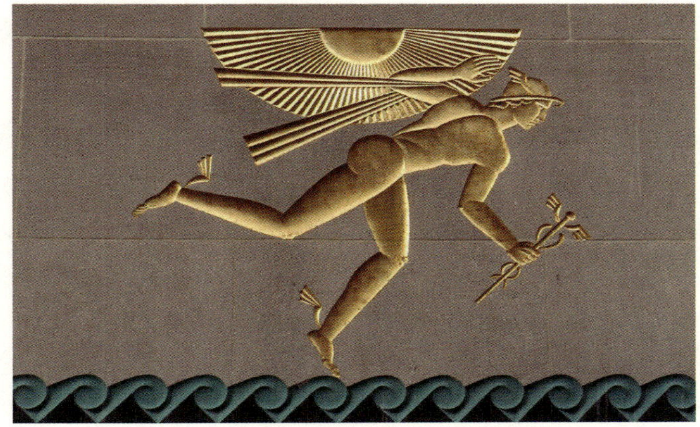

Plate 78: God Mercury with winged feet

The lung is the organ imitating the properties of Mercury. Damage of the lung during these years can alter development resulting in lifelong pathology. In another chapter we have illustrated the mesmerizing dynamic quality of this liquid metal. In its nature it resembles the dynamics of dispersion and consolidation, breath in, breath out. During the mercury period, between the age of seven to fourteen, the life body or etheric body is structured, to become an integral part of the constitution of **The One**.

The moment the secondary sexual characteristics, feminine or masculine, are manifesting the developing teenager (**The One**) is ready for a promotion so to say to a higher sphere (during sleep). Now the goddess Venus will appear in dream content and play an important role in the soul structure of the youth. She is the seducer, introducing lasciviousness; she rules over love and its compulsive sickness. She is the instigator of inappropriate behavior and socially unacceptable pranks. Her target organ is the kidney and the metal that personifies her being is the warm lustrous highly conductive metal copper. Sensing the maturing of the human being in her care, she induces (stimulates) the dialogue between opposites, and asks for reason and wisdom to make independent choices. During these seven years the astral body, the body of motion and emotion, is strengthened to incarnate, fashioning the independent personality. More and more the personal identity shimmers through in the social activity, judgments, and predilections. Although seduction is a threat, overcoming these adversities, strengthens the fiber of the personality.

Once the youth has traveled through these three spheres while sleeping, the twenty-one-year milestone has been reached. It follows out of the foregone progression that the time arrives for instructions of "I"; its strength, value, and goals are to be pursued. Only in the Sun sphere with the lofty hosts of compassion can such an education take place. At this time a discussion of these stages is not needed for further illuminations on this chapter.

Pictures out of my own biography and case histories learned from practicing in a community for over forty years can reflect truths and impress on the imagination. I am convinced that as a relative outsider, sharing my experiences with the community that has become such an integral part of my life will bring, if rightly understood, joy in recognizing some truths and meaning. Most of all it could encourage all of us to heed the inner voice, reject the skeptical naysayer and become steadfast in recognizing the inner strength that lays dormant in young and old. That is spirit! My spirit adds value and meaning to an inner reality. As a continuous stream my life flows away and only memories remain. Frankly, at no time have I ever had the experience or distinct memory of past lives. Reason and inner knowing gives me the certainty that no other possibility exists. This subjective experience is a part of my Credo. It is intimately connected to the acceptance of the Christ in my life. In my imagination He is like an Alien, the Earth preparing for him a human body to dwell in for three years. In that time span he teaches the esoteric higher life that only a handful of disciples fathom. It will certainly take more than one life to comprehend the far-reaching consequences of His incarnation. Through my actions, my will, I desire to serve Him throughout time immemorial.

The question arises: how can I serve patients who request a consultation? It will suffice to act out of my personality, my affability, and knowledge to diagnose, guide, and prescribe for them. As an individual I see the individuality of patients and must meet them in a frame of destiny that brings constructive interaction. These patients come of their own volition, or could be sent by unseen forces to work through a crisis. I often inquire about a patient's impulse to visit my medical practice. Astounding but not surprising is the frequent answer that a clue was given to them through a dream. The picture emerges in which patient, doctor, and the spiritual world act out a relationship existing over a longer period of time, through past incarnations, but also in consideration of the future.

Story of the Unbeliever

I feel impelled to introduce a story illustrating a near death experience in a brilliant individuality with a strong denial of immortality or multiple incarnations on Earth. Because of a superior power of reasoning as a researcher interested in the social and economic sciences, he often requested extensive sessions at which time we shared opinions also on the eminent thinker, spiritual investigator philosopher, and my teacher, Rudolf Steiner (1862–1925). The patient was a short, stocky man in his mid-sixties, evidently healthy with an enormous energy and focused decisiveness. He reminded me of a leader, with a familiarity in giving orders, himself living a no-nonsense, orderly life. Meeting this individuality left a lifelong impression on me, and I valued his friendship enormously. He was an individual who appreciated the world of the sense-perceptible, and who demanded discipline from the persons he worked with because he himself was a disciplined objective thinker. As a connoisseur of life, the arts as represented in literature, music, and theater had his full attention. Throughout the years of the frequent encounters, I observed a reticence in his revealing any subjective feelings concerning immortality. Like most hardcore scientists schooled in the best institutions of America, he denied the existence of experiences involving suprasensory occurrences. For him, the bodily nature was unassailable: once dead, existence was no longer. Discussions on a dual nature, personal experiences that were not in the "flesh," were easily discarded as subjective, not reproducible, and insignificant, and useless a contribution to the human sciences. Topics I was interested in discussing included such questions as: What is life? How can it leave? Where does it go? Exact science requires answers, and we faced many dilemmas wherein sensory observation and scientific investigation could not reveal the answers to us.

He did heed the existence of an inner world, evidenced in his capacity to read to his wife every evening like clockwork. Whether the text was chosen by him or her I cannot be sure. However, for a woman evaluating such activity from the outside, these are times that intimacies can blossom and be meaningful for a partnership. Such a gifted individuality must sooner or later encounter a meeting with another reality, more truthful and whole, opening the world of the spiritual kingdom beyond the already familiar three other kingdoms. This meeting came to him in the specter of the being of cancer. The medical protocol advised surgical castration to which he consented. As with the brilliant philosopher and theologian Abelard who lived in the twelfth century, this humiliating surgery was performed and changed his life in unexpected ways. The path of transformation begins here and we will start to explore this history, as an illustration to that of which a great expansive soul is capable.

My visit to the hospital was three days following his surgery. The recuperation was well within the expected parameters. The previous night, however, there was an "incident" that prompted a follow-up visit the next day. Apparently he had taken a bath, as a preparation for discharge, had fainted while rising out of the water, and hit his head against the rim causing a deep laceration of the scalp. After being given a local anesthesia the wound was stitched but his discharge was postponed for 24 hours. He was seventy-two years old. He shared with me an out-of-body experience, a separating from his body. He identified this as his consciousness, associated with his capacity to observe himself objectively, from a corner in the room. He was standing in the bathtub, but his consciousness was not "in" it. He was riveted with surprise. A blissful feeling descended in or around him, a knowing that he had completed his life, that there were no regrets or loose ends, and that now he could continue the journey that he desired to undertake. "Looking" back he saw his body crumbling, bending over, and with a loud explosive sound hitting the metal rim with his skull. It was as if this traumatic shock pulled him back into his body, overwhelming him with gravity, disappointment, and lament.

At no time during the next three weeks, the time period it took him to adjust to a rebirth coming to Earth as a different person, did I offer any opinions or insights. This was his journey and I assisted him by listening and observing the slow process of life teaching him higher realities. We know the biography of the human being divided in seven-year stages. What would take seven years in a human life, he undertook in seven days.

The first day he was incontinent and not able to stand. He could grasp objects, and was able to feed from a bottle. He became aphasic after he had shared with me his experience, a significant fact that favored the diagnosis of the patient undergoing an inner journey, in contrast to a cerebral damage from the injury. On the second day continence returned, and he was able to stand. At the end of the day he shuffled. I was at his bedside to observe. He wanted to be read to, but chose picture books. He liked flowers but not any sounds or strong odors. He sought frequent contact with the eyes but still did not speak. The third day he showed a remarkable improvement. He wanted to sit in a chair, feeding himself. His sentences were like short orders. When I came through the door he greeted me with a bright smile. His family must have valued my visits, or perhaps he ordered them out of the room. At no time was there interference in this process of healing. The wounds healed; there was no physical discomfort requiring sedatives, and his sleep was undisturbed. From the fourth day on, very slowly but deliberately his independence returned. The vocabulary had grown by leaps and bounds, his sentence structure became more mature and he started to voice opinions about local events told to him by the family. There was no interest in the enterprise he was connected to throughout his life. It was on the sixth day he had a desire to revisit the incident in the hospital. The realization that he himself had experienced a dual existence, a fact he worked on by himself in the hours of aloneness, was not easy for him to digest. At no time did he seek guidance in the spiritual sciences. His spiritual independence was at this time also a matter of pride and hanging on to a manhood that was only a memory. In his soul he was seeking and finding meaning, and adjusting to the burden of life. What do I have to live for? Not for name, not for fame, not for gain. There rises in me the need to play, and how can I project this change without upsetting family, caretaker?

There was a curious but subtle change in the second week. His body was healed, so there was no necessity for me to continue visits, but through his insistence we continued the existing friendship and played. Chess and cribbage were his two favorite past times. He always won and this irritated me to the hilt. I hate losing! But nothing was so astounding as when he opened Pandora's Box. Slowly he revealed to me in greater detail the expansive experience in the short time of what I would call the loosening of the sheaths. We referred to this as The Bathroom Scene. The tableaux of his total life experience appeared as a panorama before and around him. At that time it was a spontaneous phenomenon that awoke in him a knowing that a continuation of life was certain. Steadfast in his Self, he sensed a completion of the life on Earth, realized the duality of his inner core, and accepted immortality as the absence of death. As he described it in humorous terms: "To die is to discard the physical body, the body that has served me so well during all these years." Being the eternally inquisitive scientist he wanted to explore what that box was all about! His experience was so vivid, that the hours of focused contemplation, after The Bathroom Scene made him realize that invisible realms will open up for the self if the idea of a dual existence can be toyed with. He was literally occupied by standing and walking in a world of thought. These invisible realms, made alive again through the imagination and memory of that incident, filled him with emotions far beyond daily experiences. What became internally alive was like a Greek myth and I could play the role of the muse. The whole impression of his soul being, his strength, his rigidity, the rich characteristic structure of inheritance, was only a part of the being of two. That other part, the immortal aspect to which he was willing to concede, had as of yet no name. Was it Spirit?

His familiarity with theater, especially Shakespeare plays that he could now study intensively, helped him to identify previously unknown or rejected parts of himself. In the past, his higher Self, which I refer to as the "I," was working and organizing with a will to rule over the spirit instead of facilitating this spiritual entity to expand his world of knowing. The Spirit when taken into consideration as an entity separate from the body acquires independence of the body. He could immediately accept and "digest" this reality and the consequences that the aversion to spirit had on the evolutionary path of humanity. This diversion toward a one-sided development of powers of understanding provided by natural science awoke in him an urge to open within himself new paths of investigation. Did he have enough Time?

After three weeks we took our leave from each other. His knowing throughout the day consciousness that a duality, a spirit being and his bodily being presented itself to the world, helped him to think and accept his own immortality. The cessation of function of one part does not mean the demise of the spiritual part. The reality that eventually he would be freed from motion and emotion opened up exciting and interesting possibilities. His last words to me were, "Let us be open to learn what comes after my (death), a world where I will meet you again!" For three years all interaction between us ceased but he was good to his word. One evening he phoned to inform me of the progression of his disease. He made an inquiry as to certain medicine he had saved over the three years of his retirement. Much thinking was exchanged. Little was said. Early the next morning my eternal friend and patient came to me to say Fare Well! His presence was palpable as a space occupying force field.

There is no question about the nature of the dying process as part of The Bathroom Scene that my patient had to undergo. Excarnation is another term frequently used in Spiritual Science for the near death experience.

As was explained before, I referred you to the four sheaths or veils, as phenomena in the makeup of the human constitution. Under certain conditions such as fainting, near drowning, or poison ingestion, the sheaths around an organ or of the whole body loosens. The first sheath to separate is the denser watery entity also referred to as the etheric body or life body. In the case of total separation, the physical body deprived of the protection of its life-bestowing function and will proceed with the death process. Deprivation of Oxygen sets in motion a cascade of deathly biochemical reactions. One wonders if the combining of the atom C with the atoms N and H to form the deathly HCN cyanide molecule in the absence of oxygen could play a role.

The phenomena of experiences that occur in connection with the separation of the etheric body are described in many NDE. How many people talk about that beautiful tableau, a sum total of the memories accumulated throughout their whole life? This appears around the person in a colorful display, things long forgotten, states of vulnerability, sadness, joy, and harm perpetrated to others is now remembered through this body of memory and mercifully left behind when the individuality (**The One**) travels up and on. Most people who have experienced this phenomenon do not understand the miracle and are able to forget it quickly.

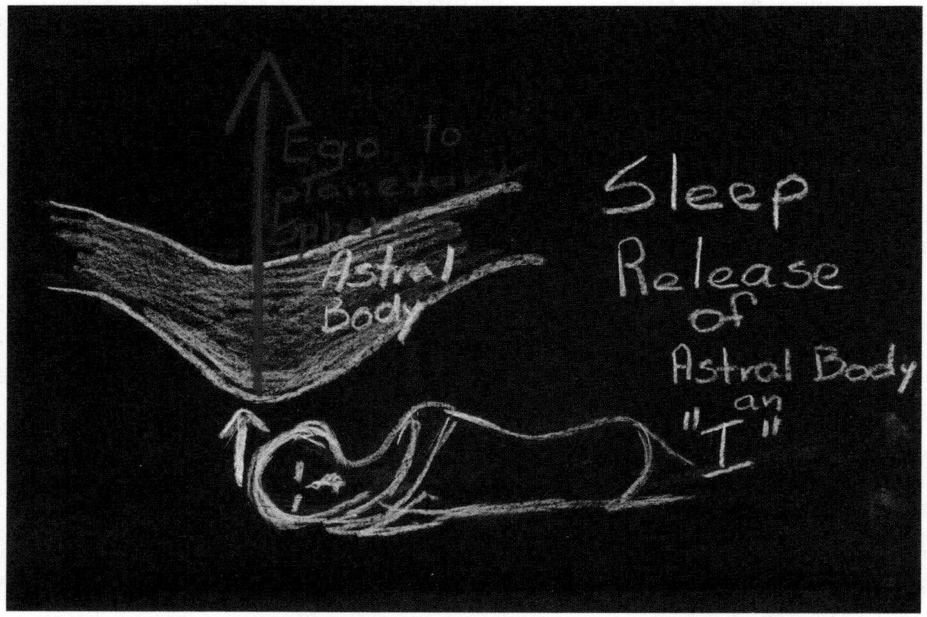

Plate 79: Sleep and separation of astral body and "I"

The reason for my patient showing a reticence in discussing it was his need to weigh the experience in his own mind. For days he was occupied with reviewing, giving careful examination, and obviously failing to find points of reference unless the existence of Spirit was considered. This indeed was no laughing matter yet in the second week he received help out of his own new constitution, mercurial as it was then, and inevitably his own fully present individuality as an eternal infinite flame was embraced.

The discussion and experience of the etheric body separating from Physical Body brings me to question if with the astral body a similar life-changing scenario can unfold. An awakened state, being aware of my surrounding with a continuous feedback from the senses can give me the impression that an unconscious life does not exist. Yet most of us are bombarded daily by negative emotions, feelings of stress, frustration, anger, anxiety, and loss of joy. In short the unknown world of passive experiences to which we have submitted. The world of the unconscious wells up through the veils of daily activity, and the astral body (as the body of emotion) experiences these hindrances. Thus the content of the astral body is not only what is remembered from the past and present consciousness, but also the part hidden in the unconsciousness. The explorations made into the hidden nature and the unrevealed aspects of the personality fall in the domain of Psychology. The submerged life of habits, suppressed trauma of childhood, and dreams are all food for analysis during therapeutic counseling by the Psychologist.

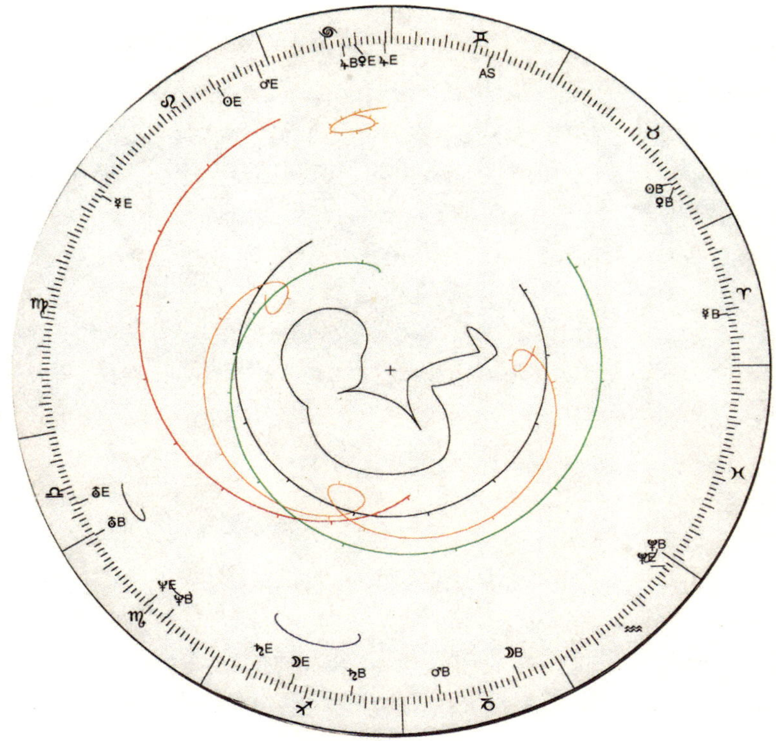

Plate 80: Zodiac belt around the fetus

During sleep the body of emotions and the consciousness there of has separated from the body. While in an induced coma no memories or dreams are retraceable, however in the state of sleep valuable information of unconscious soul hurdles are revealed to us in dreams. Carl Jung (1890–1962) a Viennese physician and psychologist, has done groundbreaking work on the psyche of the European Soul, and through his unceasing reconstruction of his own journey into his unconscious, identified the importance of the collective unconscious and Dream work. Through his numerous publications he inspired many followers by his methods in counseling who were seeking to gain a freedom from these soul restraints. The treatment protocol demanded weekly visits over years. What could be attained during these sessions? The Jungians (as this school of discipline was referred to) were not acquainted with Spiritual Science and did not adhere to the concept of the astral body. Naming this bodily sheath after the celestial spheres, which brings consciousness (emotions and willed movement) most likely connects to the sages of old. Out of antiquity we bring to modern astrology the knowledge of the Zodiacal belt, which includes the twelve segments occupying the heaven's circumference, most of which are connected with an animal name. True to the recognition in Anthroposophy, even these vast distant cosmic spaces, positioned like a belt around our solar system, have imponderable influences on the human being. The old masters still knew and assigned the heavenly regions as being the home of the creator gods, who also endowed us with the vices, hurdles in our soul-response that we will have to transform into virtues during our multiple lifetimes on Earth. Virtuous persons—those who have overcome many vices through multiple lives on Earth—can be recognized by others by walking their path on Earth as human beings who are upright, honest, loyal, without greed and jealousy, and, foremost, with love for fellow human beings and an aim toward freedom.

Throughout the ages, religious institutions have prodded humanity's conversion by advocating a style of life that imitates the "Savior." Humanity has now entered a stage of evolution in which the process of purifying the vices of the astral body will be individual conscious activity within the soul. Repetitive evening evaluations of one's own stumbles during the daily exposure of life, contributes to the cleansing process. Such a task belonged to the inhabitants of temples and cloisters. Now a process of personal awakening and desire for growth and maturation replaces the outside pressure. From the past much will be rejected. Nevertheless, the truth and knowledge of a relation with the heavens will grow stronger.

The human being as **The One** is a space-occupying body at the moment of birth, when the child takes the first breath. The position of these constellations are exact in time and space, meaning that each human being is imprinted with a unique celestial pattern in his astral body, the body equipped to receive and hold onto this cosmic reality. I marvel to think that the guidance and direction given to us from cosmic spaces is so organized that the desired virtue to be attained in an incarnation is connected with a zodiacal region (F. Julius, *The imagery of the Zodiac*). To decide the timing of birth (R. Steiner, *Eugenic Occultism*) under the guidance of cosmic forces means to choose a vice given to us through the zodiacal imprint (R. Steiner, *The Challenge of the Times* p. 103). Of course this is also the springboard for all the popularized astrologic manipulations directed by earthbound, materialistic thinking.

In the beginning after my conversion to the practice of medicine extended by Anthroposophy the understanding of the astral body was an urgent need. This body, through which emotions and movements manifest, is elusive mainly because the conventional training blinds us in believing that the personality designates the character; spiritual matters; and relationships with our ancestors, family, and friends. Study of psychiatry and psychology could not reveal the real secret behind mental disorders. Natural Science faces closed doors when the human psyche is researched; and breakthrough information again is expressed in brain enzymes, genetic disposition, and all the newest research available.

A clear distinction between the personality and the individuality is not grasped. The personality is very much a product of family, genetic disposition, religious orientation, and geographic location. For the child, these factors become the support system and imprint a future adult emotion and soul life. In a previous chapter you were encouraged to form an image of the human being experiencing a two-dimensional plane. For every person the horizontal plane refers to their role in the family, work, and society. Getting stuck in this dimension, trusting only conscious experience, satisfying impulses, and receiving affection from the world around, will not complete the factor of happiness. Facilitating the inherent soul power of thinking, feeling, and willing, the interaction between the world around me, and my own being, will take on a whole new dimension of give and take. Most human beings primarily think of themselves first. Being human with many transactions to handle during the day, I hear these words from other; "What is in it for me?" Becoming conscious of this interference is the first step of self-growth. Reviewing these thoughts at the end of the day is a mandate for developing an intense feeling life where more and more the stumbles we make become conscious reminders for correction. Only with compassion, instead of guilt, can I as a person learn to accept my personal shortcomings. With the will to embrace the rhythm of the daily review the next day will bring a change in whatever is encountered. Those short repetitive inner jolts that run like; "Who does she thinks she is?" "I feel put down!"

"I will annihilate you!" "Why her and not me?" "Nothing goes right for me." "Poor Me!" can be transformed.

On the horizontal plane our tools are thinking, feeling, and will to act. Behavioral therapy brings changes and relief to my patient, but without the introduction of the existence and ultimate recognition of the unique individuality the patient remains "unwhole," in a state of limbo.

Simply put, I have a body, I am not my body, followed by, I have a soul when thinking, feeling, and acting, but I am more than a soul function. It is staggering for me to realize how many patients seek help and become truly ill, on account of physical as well as soul imbalances. I mean by this an imbalance between our thinking, feeling, and willing; and a lack of control over the latter functions. Only through a path of Spiritual Science can I be introduced to the reality that behind the personality an individuality exists. This explains my preoccupation with these two planes—the horizontal and the vertical. The horizontal earthly dimension, an existence in time and space bound by earthly limitations, was described in the previous paragraphs. I can use my focused attention when describing the expansion into a vertical stream and identify with the concept of inner knowing. In a state of quietness when thinking is stilled or focused, an outside power flows in and meets the core of my being. I recognize existence beyond daily life. The tools of my perceiving are the transformation from my focused thinking into imagination, from feelings into inspiration, and from my will into the capacity for intuition (refer plate 25).

Silence is the conditions for opening the vertical dimension. This conversation or exchange with entities in this vertical existence, gives me the capacity to embrace Spiritual truths and the facility to unite with higher beings. The subtle embrace with the gods clarifies the saying: "It thinks in me." Suddenly I can let go of the lower self-wanting to be first, most important, and the center of attention.

The recognition that my individuality has no gender in higher spheres merging with a Totality beyond naming, and an awakening to my own duality and assignment in the earthly sphere, makes me an eternal citizen in the creation. My Higher self has an unending love, tolerance, and enthusiasm for the activity and goals I am attempting to fulfill while living my life as a human being. As a guide the world of Spirit leaves me the guardian angel, the being that protects me in my vulnerability, both physical and psychological, throughout my life. Do you have the feeling that you are watched from above? Do you have a certainty of someone keeping you out of trouble? Only in the growth of the personality while on Earth can **The One** evolve out of the state of interdependence with the Godhead and develop the urgent volition to take over the evolution and responsibility for all of humanity. The proclamation stated by Christ (John 5:10) clearly states that the human is prepared for godhood, joining the hierarchies in the unending glory of creation.

Let me revisit the Emerald Tablet, which mentions the movement of the **The One** between Earth and Heaven. It is described in postulate seven. *It ascends from Earth to Heaven, and then returns back to Earth. So that it receives the power of the upper and the lower.* The combined excarnation of the astral body, and the "I," is attained in deep meditation, during sleep, with a fainting spell, during an induced coma as in anesthesia, or after a brain injury. A state of "sleep" guarantees the visit of the "I" and astral body to the heavens.

It is comforting to know that in all these cases there is a literal ascendance to the heavenly home, an astral plane, a dimension filled with beings and regions that hopefully will protect the kernel of the vulnerable body-free existence. That is my plea for protection whenever I leave my physical and life body behind and in the care of a circumstance I am not able to control. This pendulum swinging between Heaven and Earth is possible by dent of the body-layers, their independence while existing in other dimensions, creating opposite realities humanity will eventual recognize as follows:

1) A state of forgetfulness and a state of wakefulness when memories accumulate.
2) Living in two worlds—one as the earthly dweller, one as the initiate of astral planes where other dimensions are introduced.

The earthly home is bound to time and space and requires perception and soul expression. In the heavenly home where sense activity is left behind, our instruments of experience are imagination, inspiration, and intuition. Here the declaration of the Wise One *Hermes Trismegistus*, that power is received in both worlds becomes clear. While on Earth in a wakeful state, I can develop power out of my own volition, power to will, power to control my destructive thoughts and feelings, power to do good, power to sacrifice. But once I am asleep, I will receive the knowing from a spiritual sphere, delivered to me, not out of nothingness, but in a dimension with the presence of departed souls and heavenly hosts. How many of us have received messages from departed loved ones through dreams? I can declare the power that will eventually belong to all of humanity, the power of the oneness in all. This illumination can be worked for while in the earthly dimension. Many of us know it, search for guidance, and explore possibilities, even with drug-induced states. These are examples I have explored on other pages.

Story of the Believer

In the path of healing, or acquiring a balance in daily life, the work in self-discovery has to be undertaken. Patients with a terminal disease such as cancer can decide to choose an alternative treatment that includes intense self-exploration where the "I" wills itself to find the origin of the imbalance through dream analysis. Such a patient visited Pleroma Farm, a therapeutic farm in Hudson, New York, that for seven years blossomed as a retreat for persons in search of a spiritual path in their recovery of health. My patient's process of healing becomes an illustration of how Spiritual Science can open a pathway to feel the power of "mind over matter." Her story follows.

It is amazing to realize the hundreds of hours that Carl Jung, as psychiatrist and researcher, dedicated to the unconscious, unraveling the hidden emotional life with the help of the collective stories and human dreams; addressing the imbalanced soul, or what I designate as the astral world. My patient, from whom I could learn so much, was a Jungian analyst. She was born in Canada of a father who was a blue-collar worker, and a mother who lived vicariously through this younger daughter. Our patient, now fifty-six years old was sensitive, cultured, artistic, and endowed with an extraordinary beauty and purity. The mother had dedicated herself to the dance career of this second daughter from the age of five, and did not let up until she became a ballerina. She was coerced, at a young age, to be in bondage to the compulsive dreams of a parent. She indeed became professional, later opened a ballet school, but could not find a trustworthy comfortable partner until in her late forties. She had no pregnancies. At the age of forty-nine, she was diagnosed with uterine cancer. This diagnosis was a wakeup call and the decision was made to search for a healing without the conventional interferences. Consequently major changes in her biography were registered. She left the dancing profession, followed a three-year course in Jungian analysis, accepted a guide for her own soul exploration and started an intensive discipline in dream analysis. After seven years, although her physical health was not a worry to her, a physical examination did reveal a walnut size pelvic tumor for which all modern treatment was rejected. Instead she came to Pleroma Farm, to acquaint herself with the medical practice and therapies extended by Anthroposophy. After a treatment protocol was established, the use of the remedies, injections, therapeutic eurythmy, and counseling was administered. She established a visit twice a year for seven years.

The most important work done during the first visit, which is a forty-day retreat, involves careful intensive study of the biography (O'Niell, *Human Destiny*). Every seven-year block from birth to her present year is examined. Each block is in a different light according to the journey her astral body undertakes during sleep. The experience for the patient is a plunging into a world of unknowns in which the "I" objectively unravels the dynamic interaction between herself and the family she chose for a vehicle of incarnation. She learns that the dreams now guiding her each night may reflect the intense work of memory retrieval in that stage of her life. Together the patient and the guide start to explore the feelings toward the parents. Her father was a gentle submissive man who she absolutely adored. *(The dream here was a fishing scenario. Both persons are standing on the bank of the river. He hooks a big fish and prepares a meal for her.)* Her mother, the dominant caregiver did give her the dream of dance and could make this reality come true through enormous sacrifice of her own life task. Exploring mother–daughter relationships, whereby a vicarious transference of mother over daughter is witnessed, awakens the reality that the existing pathology is intertwined with the combined feminine axis—the mammary glands and pelvic gonads. For her, it was impossible to create a distinct, strong energy around her own feminine axis, and she finally succumbed to a malignant invasion in the pelvis. Shortly after the passing of the Mother at the age of ninety-four, the patient's transition followed.

The goal in therapy for patients with an incurable disease is to expand the power of their own being. The big fish the father prepared as a meal—that is power! When I have to face the transition; "What will give me strength and power to go over the threshold?" What does give strength is when the patient can answer the questions: "Who Am I?" "What is my past, present, and future?" I gain power from knowing the impact each unique being has over me. "How will people remember me?" "What is the legend I leave behind?" "What is my unique essence that I can take as a gift for the hosts in heaven?"

For seven years the conversations during treatments continued. Physically the tumor progressed to become a stage class IV.

When her mother finally died at the age of ninety-four, permission to finalize her earthly existence was explored and finally activated. Her last gift to me was an exquisite small piece of artwork titled The Birthday.

Reexamining my experiences with her throughout the years, the question arose: "What can I remember her by?" It is this artistic jewel! I scrutinize coming to the realization only now, she knew all along her own destiny, cosmic journey and infinite existence. The certainty of accomplishment true to the beauty she was able to represent while on Earth in dance, painting, and in the social succor shared with so many human beings. Fully aware of spirit, she understood the Spiritual Sciences and traveled unencumbered in the dimensions that lay ahead of her. Here the believer becomes the knower.

The spiritual path of such an individual must include the certainty of immortality. Being a physician and understanding the medical profession very well, especially how loath we are to bring the truth of imminent "death" to the patient or the family, we make room for the help of a religious counterpart. But few of us have an understanding of Spiritual Science and the certainty this knowledge can bring to the patient. Ultimately that becomes the goal, knowing that a rest, peace, and a final expiration will come to all. When that time comes how will we embrace this? My deepest nature, as with every human being comes from above, not from the Earth. I use consciousness to direct a healing process. What are signs of healing? Is Euthanasia, an act or resolve made out of the patient's free will, an indication of healing? It still takes enormous courage and a strong will to blindly go where only uncertainties face you. Or are there no uncertainties for these individuals? These are only bare hints as to what spiritual guiding is about. When the patient and I are together I strive for the recognition of the imponderable element to assist in the struggle of seeking balance. Failure is not the return of the cancer in my patient. Failure would be, for

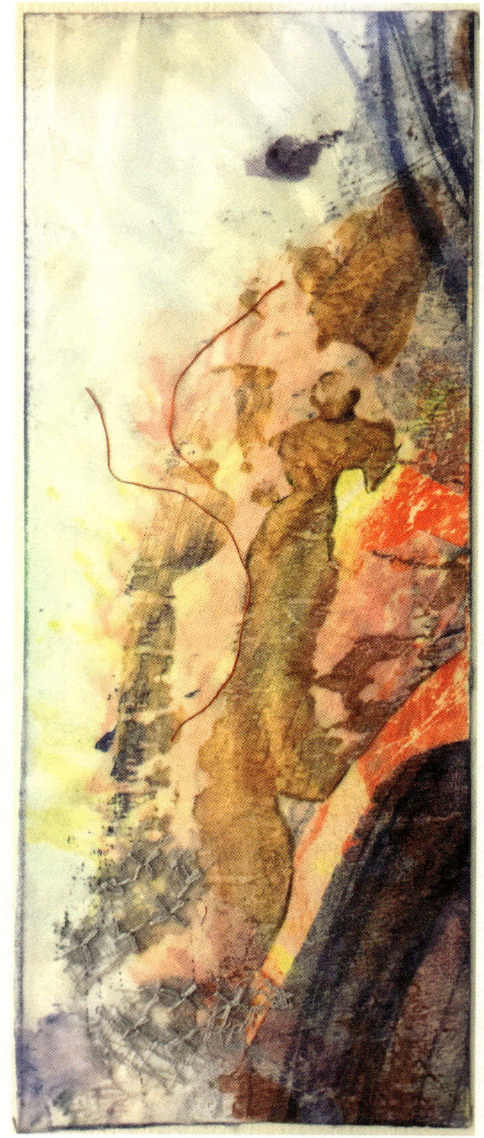

Plate 81: Birthday

example, my rejection of the patient's decision to terminate their life. Yet freedom of will and strengthening the power of **The One** is the ultimate goal of these writings.

Euthanasia will become an obstacle for the future. Today in Western medicine, especially through the practice of Hospice, the patient is assisted in dying with the help of pain medication. Suicide could be judged as an ethical issue. The family and environmental repercussions are graver then we think. Assisted suicide is legal in some U.S. states, Canada, and certain European countries. This becomes an ethical issue. The conscious will of the patient is my professional consideration. As long as I withhold my consent, I cannot assist them in the process of transition. We might all agree that **The One**, present in another dimension beyond, awaits the merging with its lower "I." The guardian protects us in our transition. Immortality is the core theme of this section in which infinite existence and reincarnation are considered. The question needs to be stated: "Is **The One** in control of its own birth and death?"

When I was young and had no consciousness of Spirit birth occurring at the same time as conception, I was in agreement with abortion. Knowing the miracle of **The One** through the study of embryo genesis, the existence of the human being before birth and the eagerness for it to experience incarnation into a material world weighs heavy on my shoulders. Pro-life should not only be a political football but an informed consent to take responsibility for **The One** and make incarnation possible. Subjectively it becomes a personal choice of the pregnant woman, a responsibility toward herself and the child's destiny. Objectively it is a matter of Law.

We end this writing with a picture given to me by one of my patients donated to my collection of *suprasensory occurrences.* Forty days after grannie's passing, this photograph of the grave was taken.

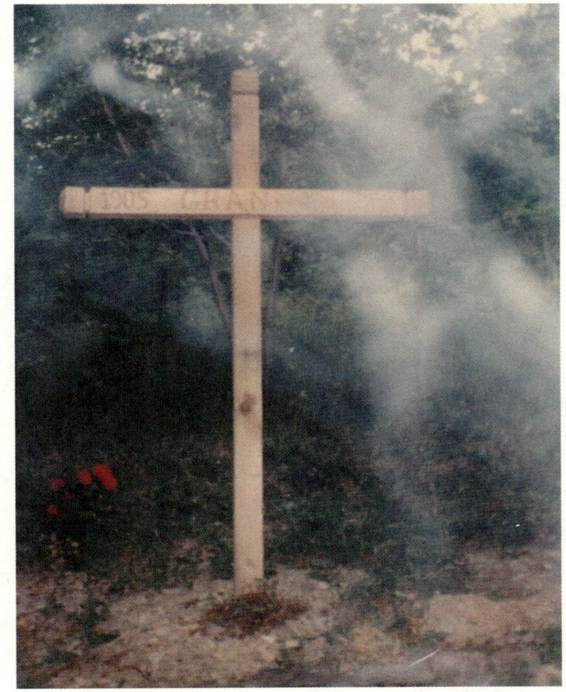

Plate 83: Granny's grave

Prometheus

Like thee, Man is in part divine,
A troubled stream from a pure source;
And Man in portions can foresee
His own funereal destiny;
His wretchedness, and his resistance,
And his sad unallied existence:
To which his Spirit may oppose
Itself—and equal to all woes,
And a firm will, and a deep sense,
Which even in torture can descry
Its own concenter'd recompense,
Triumphant where it dares defy,
And making Death a Victory.

—Lord Byron

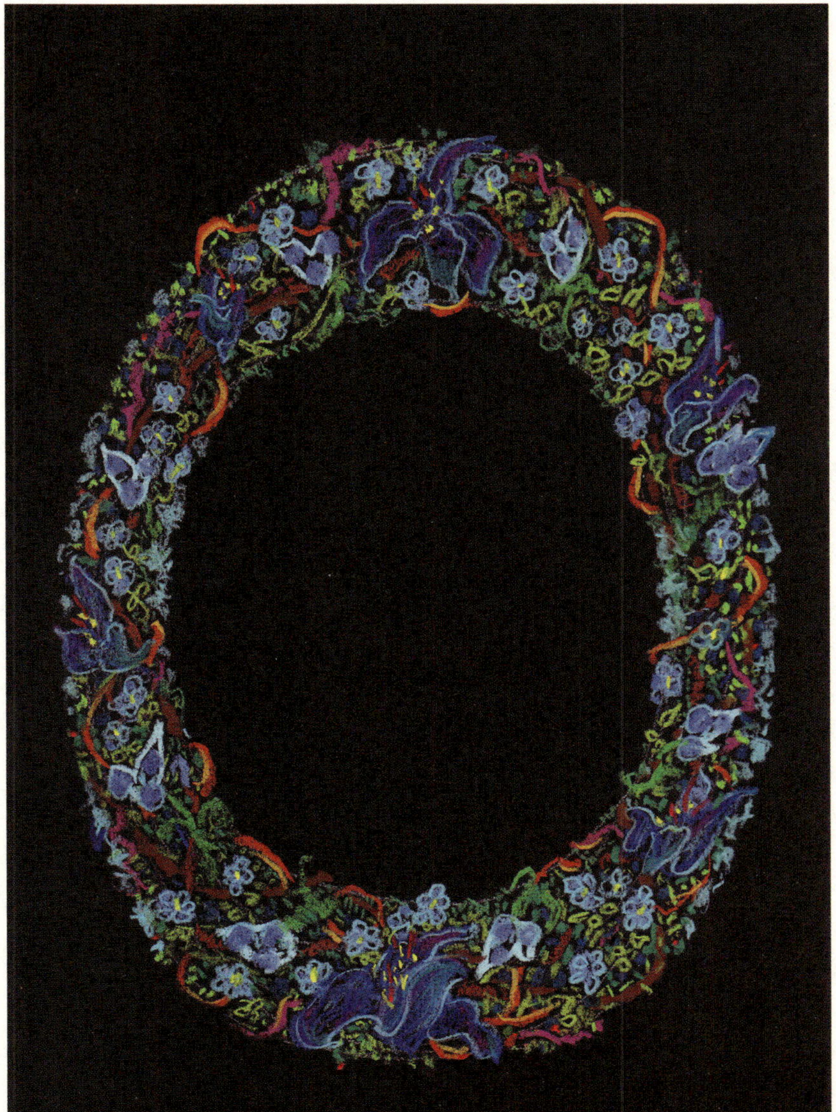

Plate 83: Sound O as depiction

Sound O

In this section the experience of the O formation in gesture and sound are examined as a testimony to the footstep of **The One** on Earth. In the sound of O **The One** learns to experience an inward gesture of containment and boundaries, self-reliance, trust in the community, and hope in the future. In the English language many words containing the O sound project an energy of comfort, inclusion but also an objective reality of aloneness. The language speaks and has a formative activity on life processes that can be demonstrated through the transformative powers of Eurythmy.

Throughout all the writings in this book, the pivotal attention is given to **The One**. The Child Artist at the age of six reminds us what our journey of earthly incarnation involves. The beginnings of existence are found in the infinite past but it is in the present that an invitation is extended for all of us to explore the essence of **The One**.

Each human being has to consider their authentic naming as the "I," which is the first step toward freedom. No one has permission to cross the boundaries of the O with which **The One** surrounds and protects itself. Out of choices **The One** makes, sharing becomes a conscious act in revealing the most intimate confessions. Confessions of past indiscretions, of personal failure but also of faith and reconciliation is an exemplary "food" for changing habitual behavior and collective destructive patterns.

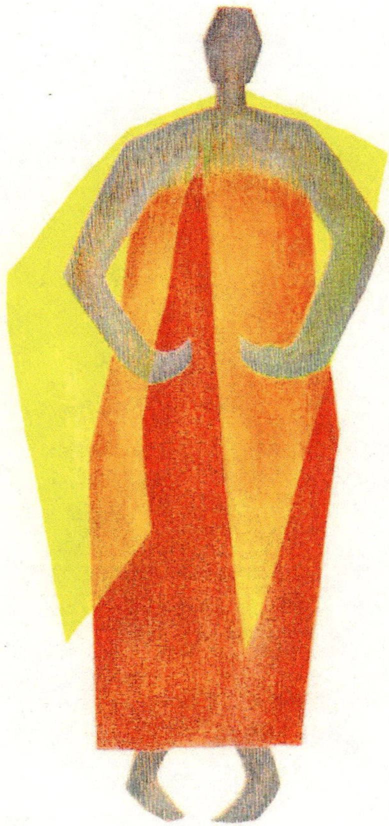

Plate 84: Eurythmy gesture of O

In today's culture and the development of the consciousness soul (Steiner, *An Outline of Esoteric Science,* pp. 46f), reintroduction to a master from the past, Hermes Trismegistus, and his the Emerald Tablet postulate, *"As above so below . . . ,"* will reconnect humanity to a needed truth for future choices **The One** can stand behind. We learn anew that the confluent streaming from above toward **The One** is a reality.

The personal path through the seven-year periods, the role of woman, mother, doctor, and lover, are all intimate O experiences that become a part of one's biography and a testimony to authenticity. This section gives examples of how human being can each attend to themselves in an earthly biography as **The One**—a member of humanity. Objective recognition of **The One** is in seeing the "other." Subjective recognition of **The One** is identifying one's own individuality.

The physical body must become an obedient instrument for **The One** working in and through it. The constitution of the human body is subject to a continuous change in structure during the cycles of the day, the month, and year, and as we know in the seven-year cycles a totally renewed cell structure manifests itself. The purification, refinement, and detoxification of physical substances are organic processes assigned to Alchemical Science, a school of knowledge now replaced by the name of biochemistry. Understanding Alchemy as it was introduced in section A, could develop an imagination wherein these processes are pictured as a continuous activity in our interior, so that the concept of self-healing could be embraced as an integral part of bodily activity. An example would be for instance a body responding with high fever as a mechanism to burn out the invasion. The concept of self-healing is of great significance because of the power of trust that is given to **The One** who chooses to assert such freedom in its own life.

The One needs to conceive its soul as an organ. Evolutionary development is assigned in mounting steps from sentient, intellectual to conscious soul capacities throughout thousands of years of world history. The soul activity of **The One** as a representative of humanity is limited to two conscious experiences (Steiner, *The Wisdom of Man*, p. 67). The capacity to reason belongs to the human soul only. At an early age **The One** is guided to judge between opposites—for instance, the *yes* and the *no*. Challenges and choices foster growth in the organ of the soul. A spontaneous capacity for love and hate is a purely human experience and becomes the second attribute of the human soul (ibid.). Through the presence of the organ of soul **The One** experiences desire and can react impulsively on stimuli arising either from conscious or unconscious in-streaming. Embroidering with these two capacities love/hate and reason, the soul as an independent emoting entity receives stimuli from two sources.

First one recognizes that perceptions through the sense organs are a continuous source of stimulation for the soul and "bombard" the exterior border of the soul organ, even during sleep. The organs of the senses are not a part of the soul but impact the soul-life continuously. On one side **The One** has to deal with the sense impressions that contribute a great deal to the content of its soul-force. From an interior place deep within or beyond this organ arises an impulse of desire that flows and mingles with the outer impressions to create a soul constitution totally unique for the personality of **The One**.

Desire rises up from deep regions of soul to meet the reality of opposites stimuli, the polarities present in the world. Light or dark, warm or cold, wet or dry, silence or noise are all conditions stimulating the senses, creating perceptions that in turn inundate the boundary present between the outside and interior worlds.

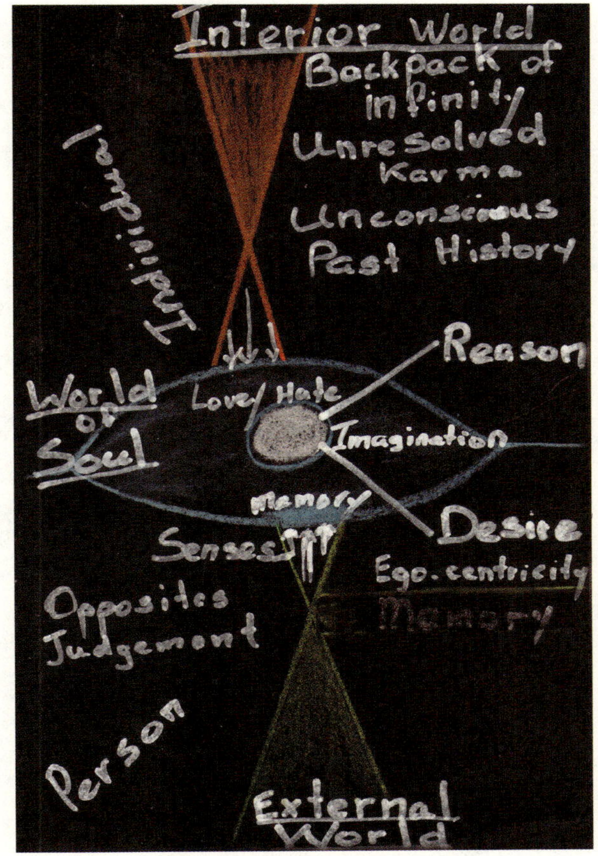

Plate 85: Soul as an organ

Steeped in such controversy, the soul experience must represent a "*battlefield upon which struggles are in progress*" (Steiner). Guidance in childhood becomes a responsibility toward **The One**'s expression of a life of desire, frustrations, controversy, as well as feelings of love and wonder. These need to be recognized in the child-being by adults. The percepts created by the sense organs, be it a sound, an image or an odor are registered by the soul-organ and create a memory. Memory formation is a secondary reaction to percepts streaming from the outer world through the boundaries and become a part of the inner soul-experience. Memory is not a soul function. It is created by the world of senses.

The force of reason, solely as a human activity, becomes the second pure soul function next to existence of attraction or rejection. Although visual perception is not a function of the soul, the capacity for visualizing images conjured up by dent of reason remains a pure unadulterated soul element.

The One identifies with a life task only with full maturation after the age of twenty-one. As a personality, manifesting at the beginning of sexual maturation, the interaction with the environment, projection of physical and emotional capacities, and recognition of talents and habits, human-beings are not authentic masters of themselves but are captivated by impulses coming from the environment and social surroundings. After the age of three times seven, with the birth of the "I" at twenty-one an interior force presents itself, a force that identifies the "I" as a separate entity. This awakens **The One** to ideologies it wants to pursue, and enables life tasks to become identified. Here the exercise of writing a Credo will be helpful (end of chapter). To reason, to use the power of deduction, to exercise the logic in the development of questions, to experience the light and triumph of the higher purpose of humankind is an inherent quality of the soul spurred on out of higher regions. Here the soul is used as instrument of execution while incarnated on the Earth. **The One** as a representative of humanity is functioning in its individuality!

The soul, as a derivative of the human being, represents one part of the trinity (spirit, soul, and body) and is, so to speak, juxtaposed between Heaven and Earth. On the Earth the life of desire finds its activity, which is expressed by the person in reactions to outer life. From higher regions an eternal aspect of the human is represented in its capacity to identify its own individuality through reason and the examination and or practice of a religious discipline. Why?

Throughout life, human beings are imbalanced in soul activity; in other words, there is dissociation among the three expressions of thought, feeling, and will. Often chaotic disturbing thoughts overwhelm our daily tasking. The experience of pain, sadness, or fear play into a soul discomfort attributed to this imbalance. The will effort is too weak to dominate the incongruities of the companion soul functions, feeling and thinking, which in turn causes discomfort. This hinders the personality in bringing to full expression the authentic self on Earth, its purpose, its connection with humanity, and the desire to maintain and remember one's divine origin. Maybe, through a religious discipline, one can gain a connection. This is only a bare hint of what wants to become spiritual. To unite with the divine is the most intense experience that the soul can attain. Have many Earth dwellers succeeded in reaching this state? There are testimonies of postulants, in both the East and the West, of searching and at times approaching a "heaven," being "surrounded by Sublime White Light," of "Ecstasy," or of rest in the Heart of God—in other words, consciousness in which all is encompassed in ONE. Experiencing Light and Bliss is objective. Naming God is purely subjective.

The Emerald Tablet reminds us of the inevitability that all **The Ones** will ascend from the Earth to a higher reality. So we can question: What is such a journey's timespan? Are there schools "up there"? What will we learn? Why ever come back? To glean knowledge to these questions means to study Spiritual Science. Researching and finding answers for the inquisitive mind has always been possible—first in the Schools of Tibet, later in the temples of Babylon, Egypt, and Greece. Most of humanity was not allowed to lift the veil of spiritual truths because the knowledge remained occult. With the end of Kali Yuga the time of secrecy has ended and humanity stands on the threshold of discoveries free to be revealed.

These truths are the essence of **The One**:

1) Immortality: after excarnation (death) the journey through the solar system begins. In each sphere dismemberment of memories occurs as they are left "behind";
2) Reincarnation: insight into multiple earthly lives, an introduction to past as well as future lives on Earth.
3) Creative progress for the human being to an ultimate perfection, executed by the hierarchies, in the likeness of the Godhead;
4) Spiritual Evolution: human beings develop the capacity for Love and Freedom;
5) Metamorphosis: changes in the physical human body to accomplish these goals.

This very much stipulates a future journey in which schooling will be necessary. All information obtained regarding the expansion of our spiritual being in celestial spheres does not come from books or religious institutions or, for that matter Earth. Within all of us there is a knowing.

The Child Artist knows and leads us. He remembers his tutelage in the heavens. I cannot do other than listen and share this information with the reader. As we have noticed from the Child Artist's drawings, there is a considerable knowing connected to the embryonic development. Cells are directed in a dance, currents of dynamic activity of restrain or deployment, choosing functions and moving to positions in the small organism where optimum responses create form and function. The one who is doing the directing is the embryonic incarnating being, **The One**.

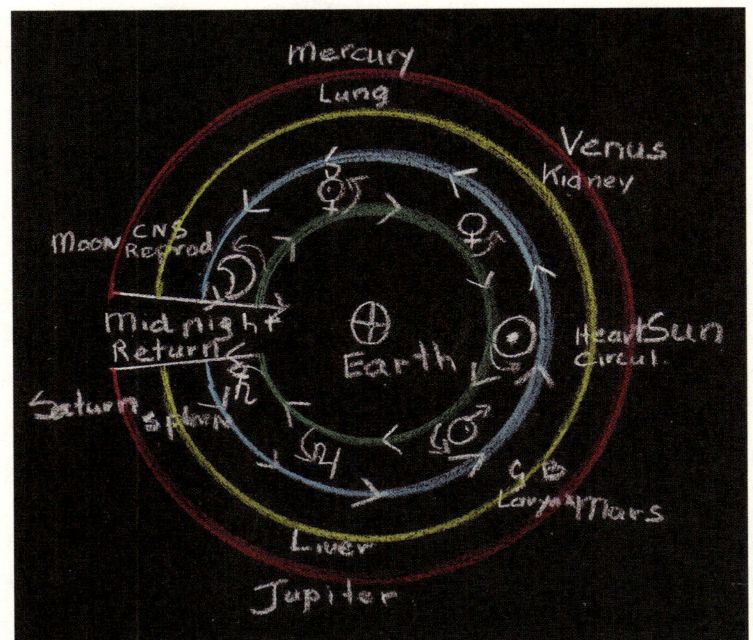

Plate 86: Leaving behind karma in each sphere

In death we part with the restrictive earthly body. The journey through our universe can be undertaken in a similar path as the journey the human being undertakes during sleep. There is a visitation into the spheres of Moon, Mercury, Venus, Sun, Mars, Jupiter, and Saturn successively until at the end we dwell in the bosom of Saturn. Imagine that the hierarchies on these celestial bodies are occupied with nothing else but expanding the understanding of the individual. This understanding of functions and form is connected with the physical body and the soul. We receive an exchange from each sphere according to the organs we fashion. For example, the Moon gives us knowledge of brain and reproductive organs. The next sphere of influence is represented by Mercury, a powerful impulse to the formation of the lung. Venus exerts influence on the kidney system formation and does interfere with the gender issue. Our circulatory system combined is placed under the dominating influences of the Sun. Mars, and beings thereof, teach us on the use of the voice through the larynx and the dominant role of the bile in digestion. The beings in the Jupiter sphere know the domination of the water content regulated by the largest organ the liver. The Saturn sphere concludes the ring of planetary existences in our solar system with its forces influencing the spleen in the rhythms of digestion and our physical body. The spleen system is physiologically little understood, and may play a more important role in future body transformation.

The Experience in O for a Person on Earth

In the sound of O the commonality of all humanity will be celebrated. Each one of us as a personality has a place on this Earth. True none of us are similar. Gender distinction and a genetic disposition we have chosen, combined with a specific time of incarnating in the last century that meets the needs to express ourselves in a challenging world of opposites. Standing figuratively speaking in a circle, holding hands so to say, expresses the willingness to accept differences, nay even welcome those humans on Earth whose habits can teach us tolerance and perseverance.

Even the agnostic person has a Credo. A person needs to identify with one's background, understand the opportunities offered by the environment, and through education know their personal potential and limitations so that the world can be influenced and changed for the better. The credo becomes a confession of the faith one has combined with an undying dedication to this reality.

The contact we have with suprasensory worlds is of yet subjective and does not make one superior as a person. What becomes outstanding in a biography is the person's recognition of vices and the steps that are undertaken to metamorphose these negative energies into something positive—namely, the virtue connected but now the opposite from the vice. The strength of self-help groups (AA) can be found in the community gathering around all those in need with the declaration and confession of helplessness and compassion. "There but for the Grace of God, go I." Only with the utmost discretion of the participants can trust be built—trust that all the persons living, working, and playing together deserve. The energy of an O gesture becomes stronger with the acceptance of differences in each person. Each person is unique, thank God! The asset of each and every one lends beauty to the tapestry we weave. A person can emulate but not imitate. There is a world of difference between those two concepts.

Gender

I want the reader first of all to understand that the gender differences are real and are explained in the following discussion that illustrates anatomical and physiological but also a soul distinction between the male and the female person. Knowledge all need to acquire as **The One**. As for myself I questioned the impact my role as a female physician had on my surroundings.

It is remarkable that the gamete as the male and female reproductive cells is prepared long before fertilization with only half of the chromosomes so that, in the process of fusing, the expected forty-six chromosomes are present. The male gamete (spermocyte cell) carries fifty percent XY and fifty percent XX chromosomes. The sperm determines gender when a XX–XX merger will develop a female body, and XX–XY male body.

All living human cells are penetrated or suffused with the etheric body, which has the capacity to exert formative forces on processes of life. Is there a distinction found in living formative forces between the male and female organization? Yes, and that is partly why I want to explain the differences more in depth. As we can deduce from foregone texts, nature's activity finds its order in fourfold adherence to the elements of warmth ether, light ether, chemical ether. and life ether. They are referred to as formative forces. Each of these four forces has distinct characteristics (Ref: *Embryogenesis and Fourfolding*). In the warmth ether and light ether we find centrifugal, radiating out, qualities. These two ethers are actively productive, transmuting substances and life affirming. In contrast the chemical and life ethers have centripetal tendencies, absorption with a tendency to embrace or enclose within them in an O gesture, reflecting an indolence and water retaining quality.

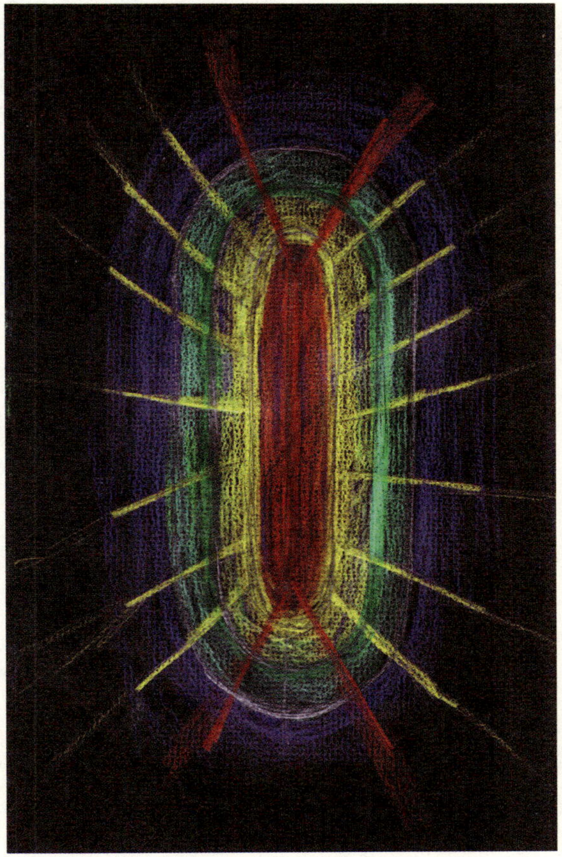

Plate 87: Cellular penetration with the life forces

The feminine with this distinct nature tends to be portrayed as passive receptive. We can deduct that these two distinct opposite qualities will have a designation in the gender psychology of the human being. It is easy to think, Men are from Mars; Women are from Venus. Let us see if this distinction has a leg to stand on!

In our understanding of the sleeping body, two distinct entities are dealt with. One is the solid corporal structure and the other the life asserting and imponderable flow of forces in all living tissues.(Also referred to as living water.) The forces occupied with the corporal structure are, as with the differentiation in the sexes, diametrically opposed. The physical difference between a male and female is undeniable. What the sexes in their psychological activity are endowed with, is, in these modern times not so clear. First the formative forces, as in the case of the gamete, split up with warmth and light ethers functioning in one pole and the chemical and life ether exacting their influence in the other pole of the body, in this case the head pole and the genital pole. The male genital pole adheres to the formative forces of the warmth and light ethers. There it exerts its true nature of activity, enthusiasm to burst out, impregnating the surroundings. The female genital pole attracts the opposite formative forces, those of chemical and life ether, and becomes preoccupied by the passive receptive formative forces.

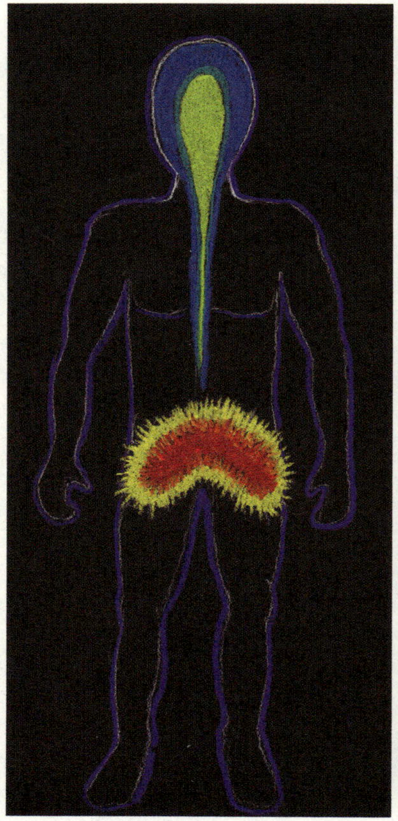

Plate 88: Polarities of the pelvis vs. head of male

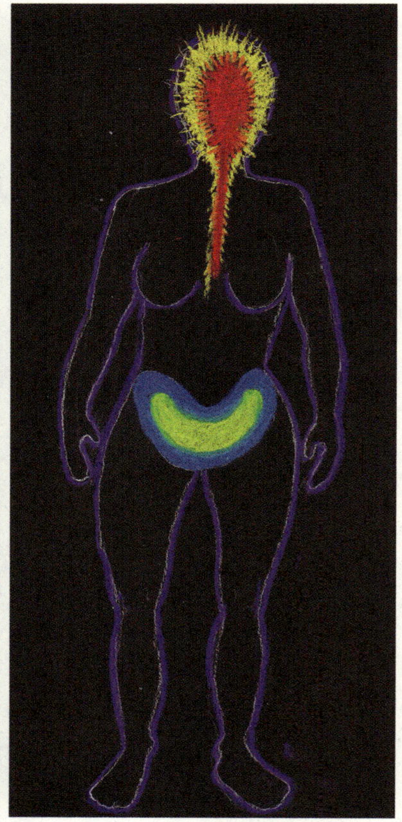

Plate 89: Polarities of the pelvis vs. head of female

Laws in nature confirm that those formative forces of the etheric body not applied to the maintaining of the corporal structure are used to assert influence on the opposite pole, the head. *That what is not used as formative force in the corporal function within the organism will serve as free forces yielding a psychological and spiritual influence on the thought processes of the person.* The spiritual and psychological function arising out of the free-flowing formative forces stimulate the head region of the two genders each in a specific way. The head-forces in the male differ from those in the female. Subjectively, as a female I have discovered throughout life that my thought processes are distinctly different from those of the opposite sex. The female can draw on the free-flowing formative forces arising out of the light and warmth ether. At her disposal is the flamboyant imagination, and an active spiritual preoccupation. Within her head new ideas are formed. She creates the future world, she becomes the muse.

On the contrary the male thought processes activate access to free-flowing chemical and life ether. Throughout the evolution of humanity the pride of the male is contained in science. In the soul of man, knowledge is his second nature. Being a scientist, he collects factual elements of knowledge. Through this embracing function being present in his head, he gathers

Fourfold in the Etheric Body

Color	Quality	Element	Flow	Corporeal Pole	Force Flow
Red	Warmth	Fire	Centrifugal	Male Genital	Female Head Pole (CNS)
Yellow	Light	Air	Centrifugal	Male Genital	Female Head Pole (CNS)
Green	Tone/ Chemical	Water	Centripetal	Female Genital	Male Head Pole
Blue	Life	Mineral	Centripetal	Female Genital	Male Head Pole

innumerable individual phenomena out of the external world (ref. C. Darwin, *The voyage of the Beagle*). Such knowledge is receptive and not creative.

In the biography of each one of us the male and female realities need to be understood, be respected, and enable us to reach out to each other. The synthesis of the masculine and feminine etheric forces is the ultimate act in the recognition of the divine nature of human beings and creation and, by uniting these etheric forces concentrated in the upper pole for spiritual action and in the lower pole for reproduction, cosmic union can be attained, giving humanity the strength and joy to create. (*This also leads to understanding the fact that humanity will eventually do away with gender distinction, again becoming androgynous in nature.*)

Sex, Love, and the Future of Humanity

Sexuality means being sexual, which in turn has several meanings varying from "having sex," to the merging of male and female germ cells, not to mention the values we personally connect to these words inspired through thoughts, fantasies, memories, or desires. In other words, sexuality is a simple word that means a lot to us. Although compared to the amount of time we dedicate every day to our job, to childcare, or to recreation, the time that we are actually sexual, meaning in this context, having sex, is relatively short. Few days pass, however, in which we do not have thoughts, fantasies, feelings, or wishes in which sex plays the central role. Sexuality, eroticism, and its derivative pornography pervade deeply enough into our existence that it justifies the question: What does sexuality mean to me, and what do I want to do with it?

One thing is clear; sexuality and love seem to be related. Then what is love? Plato remarked that the more we know, the less we understand. With love, that certainly seems to be the case. Rudolf Steiner pointed out that human beings are spirit, and their world is the world of spiritual beings (R. Steiner, *Anthroposophical Leading Thoughts*), directing us toward the insight that, if we overcome the thought forms that limit the content of our thinking to thoughts regarding the sense-perceptible world, we will graduate into perceptions of beings, which our eyes, ears, touch, and smell cannot perceive. He speaks here of the angelic beings, the hierarchies from Angels to Seraphim (R. Steiner, *An Outline of Esoteric Science*). Awareness of these beings brings us closer to understanding the future of humanity: to bring into the realms of the angelic beings qualities that only humans are able to develop. The conscious evolution of the human ability to love is intimately related to this future. Life offers us many opportunities through which we can hone our ability to love willingly. Sexuality is obviously one of these opportunities.

To understand this, one can take a closer look at what actually takes place when we have sex, or better, make love. The German psychiatrist Wilhelm Reich, MD (1877–1957), who later in his life immigrated to the United States, did extensive studies of the psycho-physiological basis of the coital act. In his book, *The Orgasm Reflex* (1923), he develops the idea that at the basis of the coital act between two people lies an energy cycle of stimulation and orgasmic relief. Excitation and building up of tension, are followed by a sudden release: the orgasm, and then relaxation. It was his understanding that this cycle is a natural and rhythmically reoccurring life process, inherent to the human organization.

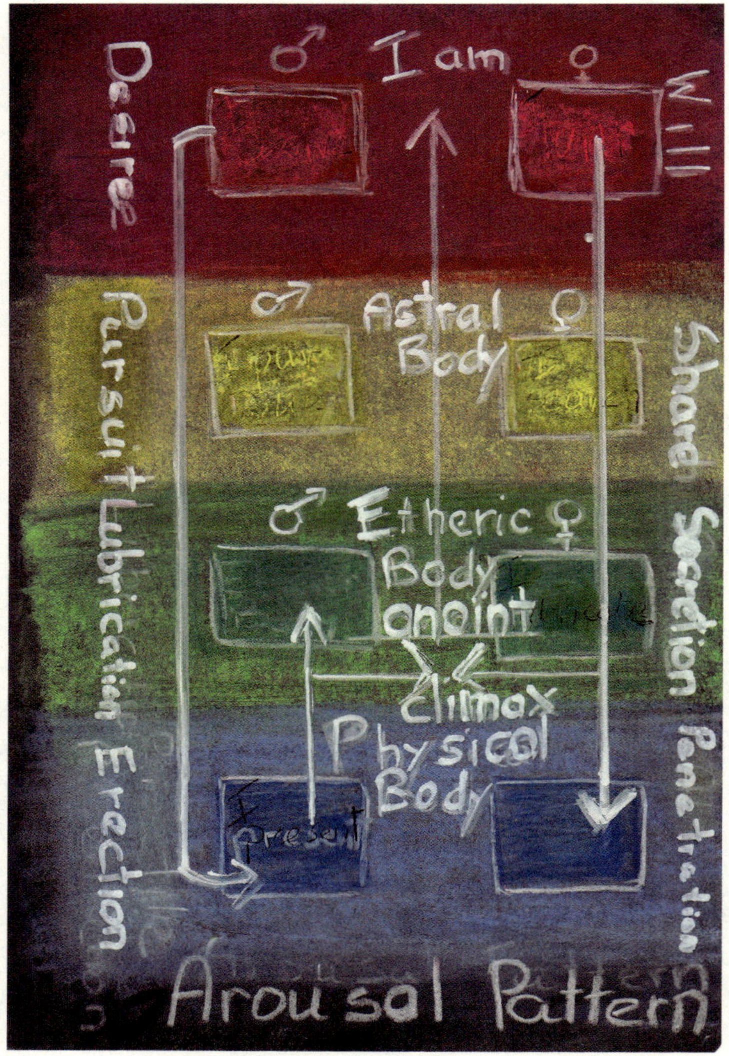

Plate 90: Gender differentiation in the pattern of arousal

There is a distinct difference in the arousal pattern between the female and male. In a living physiology that Spiritual Science can provide, subtler bodies and their function and relationship with the elements of water, air, and fire are recognized. The divergence in the response to sexual stimulation can be experienced as a pathway through these bodies (etheric body, astral body, and the Self, or "I"). Male stimulation often is physical in so far that it has an immediate effect on the genital tissue. The erectile response does not imply that the male partner is ready for the intimate sexual act. Reaching out to his partner who experiences another pathway toward readiness is an integral part of the foreplay. The feminine response follows a different path. The meeting of a being that is on the same wavelength with her stimulated "I." This state is then followed by an active fantasy in which her pleasures of touching and sharing herself with a partner arise out of her astral body. An intensification of the play causes her to have a response of her etheric body (lubrication) finally to result in readiness for penetration. The male partner has participated in his partner's process through patience and responsiveness and experiences a heightened excitement through his etheric body and his astral body, an excitation that goes far beyond only a physical acting out.

We recognize that the life process of orgasm is only one aspect of making love. Granted, our urge to have sex arises out of our physiological organization; the actual act, however, can bring us into an enormously intimate encounter with the "I," the unique, eternal being of our partner. And it is the "I" in both partners that actually directs the course of the sexual act, guiding feelings of affection and tenderness and a sense of trust toward the other as the sexual tension builds up. Toward the heights of this cascading process of mutual approach between two partners, no contradictory impulses exist.

Consciousness is turned toward the streaming sensations of pleasure. Pleasures that are distinctly different for male and female. She absorbed in the preparation to receive and embrace the male, he loses himself in her welcoming warmth as he penetrates. Then, as the involuntary orgasm approaches, the lovers lose all interest in their surroundings, absorbed as they are in their own sensations and those of their partner. The orgasm produces a loss of consciousness of one's surroundings, creating the state in which the lovers can meet each other in their true form—not perceivable to the senses. It is in this moment, when the two lovers meet in the timeless space that is created by the release, that we can receive our partner in the temple of our heart.

Here then takes place an act of love, done out of free choice, enabling our partner to thrive in earthly life, because he or she feels loved. The sexual cycle has delivered us onto a plain where we can choose time and again to open up our hearts for the "I" of the partner, making a home for this "I" in our own being. Then, relaxed we compose, thrilled by the past experience, slowly regaining awareness of life around us. Finally we walk away from the scene, inspired to recognize in our partner, as daily life shrouds one's purity, the "I" toward which our love flows.

An evaluation of my own gender placement in a foreign society, in which I became totally assimilated, permits me to ask questions on the role I occupied in this rural area. Have I as a mother, teacher, and as professional in this society, tried to share my best with the female children born in the latter part of the twentieth century? What example have I demonstrated to young women that they can emulate? How deep is the anger toward the male gender of humanity and vice versa? Am I doing the child a favor by proscribing masculine and feminine connotations to social activities? Could one trace a correlation between failed partnerships while in the role of parents, to this deep-seated mistrust and anger? These questions are collective, born out of the uncertainties of the times. To know who I am in my own being may help others. Willing to share these intimate life issues, I have written essays on the following subjects.

Being a Woman

Shortly after my thirteenth birthday I started to become aware of my body. Not only concerns about not always feeling well and energetic, but also joy and awe in the changes that inaugurated a new phase in my life, the ripening into womanhood. Discovering hair growth in intimate places, and later the first menses were also occasions for a very personal celebration. It was empowering to realize that the designation of woman made me a part of a sisterhood and I shared a special gift of reproduction. After all I was exposed to cultural mores in a restricted schooling and society of the late forties, a milieu in which intellectual development played a major role. Motherhood was believed to be restrictive and a sacrifice. Study came first.

As a child there existed an aching antipathy for my small female body. Feelings of deficiency, hopelessness in not being able to affect the world as a man, hovered around me in my own search for an identity. With an assertive disposition it was unavoidable to be teased and reminded that such behavior is not acceptable in a female. Once I was inaugurated by the natural process of ripening, my body became a part of nature, submitted like clockwork to the lunar type rhythm within. Emotional instability, bodily discomfort, and restrictive activity became stumble blocks in

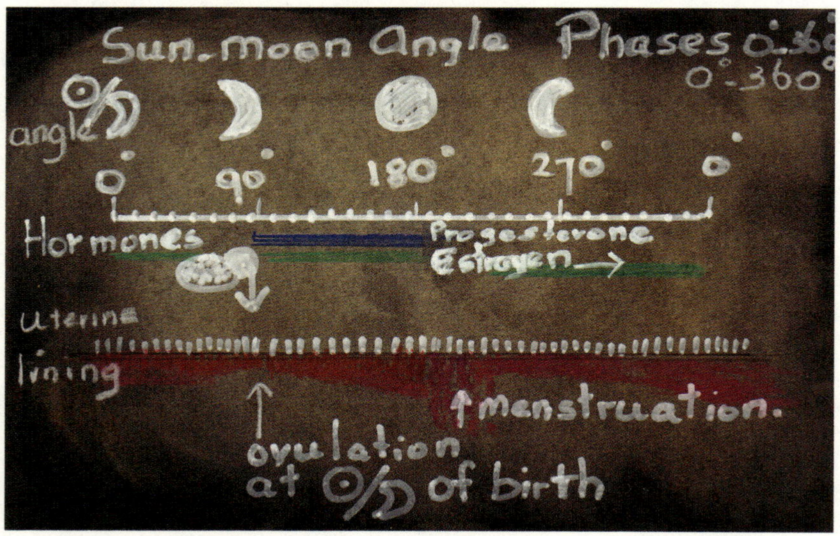

Plate 91: Three phases of hormonal secretion

my life. It is in the acceptance and understanding of these hurdles that womanhood can become a distinct affirmative aspect in one's life to explore.

To prepare the uterus for receiving the fruit of conception, there is a fluctuation in hormone levels throughout the monthly cycle. This means that the woman accedes to experiences that are foreign to her male counterpart. The presence of the ovarian hormones Estrogen, Progesterone, and changes in the levels of these two throughout the cycle creates different somatic symptoms and psychological conditions. The target for these occurring changes is the uterus. Three distinct phases within the monthly cycle can be discerned.

In the Estrogen phase after menses, the up building of the uterine lining begins as preparation for the implantation of the fertilized egg. The period after menses I would declare as being in a pure state, experiencing myself balanced between the two polar excesses I still will face in this cycle. I am free from bodily interferences. At this time only the hormone Estrogen is produced mainly by the ovary and its circulation in my body is influencing the decision-making process. The effect of this hormone on my feeling life is decisive. I feel comfortable in a state of planning. I seek validation as a compassionate being, reaching out toward the sick and tortured. I feel misapprehended and lost when surrounded by the hateful attitudes produced by the male hormone (testosterone) behaving humans. Voicing concerns for the child, the poor, the weak, and indisposed is a social response to my interior biological nature. I become an effective voice for the trodden humanity.

In the next phase, estrus has taken place. The ovary releases the ovum, and the dome of the cyst closes. The second hormone Progesterone is excreted by the remnant cystic cavity. These two hormones Estrogen and Progesterone, circulating through my body change my disposition. I become influenced by warming smoldering fire-like energy that renders me receptive and introspective. My body starts to accumulate more fluids and awareness of the breasts and pelvic organs dominate the consciousness. I can interpret this phase as carrying within myself an axis, an imaginary median presence of fecundity reflected in the area over my heart and breasts, down to the navel area and radiating into the pelvic and vulva area. The lusciousness of my being creates a social geniality that invites others to partake in my overabundance. I can woo my partner with my openness and receptiveness. In the social life I become the hostess. At my work I can arbitrate and intercede when a crisis exists. I can solve problems using my feminine wile. This is the strength of the lower pole in the genital axis drawings of the three phases

In the third phase both hormones stop to produce for a few days, resulting in the breaking down of the uterine lining and its expulsion. If an unfertilized egg is present this is also discarded. The menstrual bleeding provides the female body with an opportunity to purify the blood, the reason for the woman to be named "unclean" in this phase. In this phase of low hormone levels, profound psychological changes overpower me. This is the time when, with friends and/or colleagues, I experience the capacity for intense philosophical conversations, brilliant illuminated thought processes, and an amazing quality for understanding the evolving human condition. This is the strength of the upper pole of the genital axis. In the monthly cycle this experience becomes

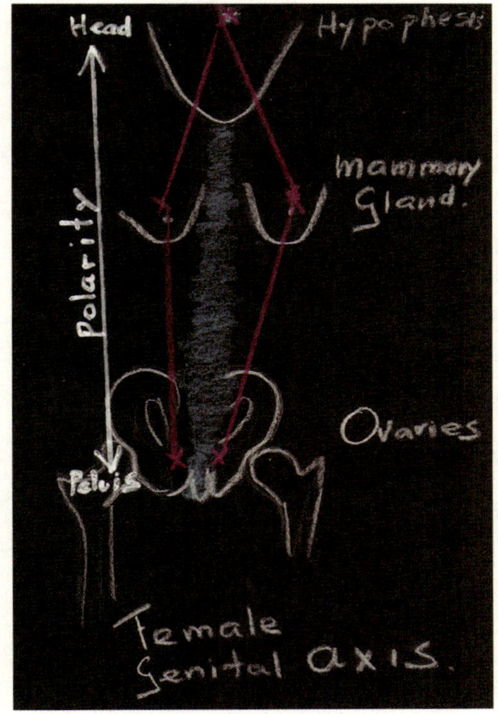

Plate 92: The female genital axis

a gift to me and creates a yearning for an indefinite continuation. When the physiological response of hosting a new life has failed, the individuality witnesses a profound source of moral inspiration available to her.

Within me I carry this genital axis—the axis of Love. The upper pole, the mammary glands, is shadowed by the upper arms capable of both embracing and warding off that what comes toward me. This pole also embodies the head organization with the capacity for clear thinking and creating moral thought. The lower pole is found between the mighty thighs. These pillars of strength surround the vulnerable feminine entrance to protect from attacks and violation.

Four thousand years ago in the time of a flourishing Egyptian civilization, the mighty temple of Luxor was build. This Temple has also been presented as the image of the human body (Schwaller de Lubitz, *The Temple of Man*). During a visit to Egypt in 1993, extraordinary experiences fructified my imagination. The Holy of Holies, the inner sanctum in the back of the Hall surrounded by strong pillars, reminded me of the feminine anatomy. Imagine rich curtain hangings representing the outer aspects of the genital anatomy, the vulva and vagina, protecting the small entry door, through which only the High Priest was permitted to enter on specific days of the year. The area was shrouded in secrecy, however I am convinced that fecundity, and the invitation of the descending spirit beings into the population was an essential part of a cult. A small room adjacent to the inner room is occupied with representations of The Pharaoh, with an enormous phallic structure placed over the navel. Out of this organ an abundant ejaculate flows forth. In those times the soul of humanity was in need of direction from the Theocracy. The Priests directed the male population regarding the humanizing of the sexual act. Those were the times shortly after the Priestesses were replaced by masculine power. Was the time for the prominent female role in the evolution closed? Did the woman respond to her own biological physiology?

Once the productive phase has ended (menopause) and the ovaries start to atrophy and hormone levels diminish, it becomes a time for enormous adjustments. Withering of the female endocrine organ in the body is experienced by waves of pouring out bodily heat followed by profound perspiration. How can these discomforts assist me in the next phase of my life? If I do not reject this phenomenon but welcome each "flush" I can cultivate the organization of my own warmth. Radiating warmth heals the ailing me so that I can find a way to stimulate social wisdom and compensate for the rejection I encounter by the society around me.

When young, using these different windows of experiences delivered to me by my internal hormonal system and the genital organs becomes a huge advantage in the understanding of the human being as we evolve toward love and freedom. As a Woman I have the opportunity to experience many talents within myself that can benefit a society faced with cataclysmic changes. As I enter the phase of the crone, wisdom develops by leaps and bounds. I dare to follow my heart and attend to latent capacities. I continue to grow.

The correlation between the Feminine as represented in humanity and in the universe exists. Take heed and listen! Gaia our beloved Earth is wounded. Her body is scarred by wartime craters. Through deforestation her breathing is impaired. Nature as her garment is torn and tattered. The final blow is the dictum "Axis of Evil" politically created in an act of denial that She even exists. As a human proclamation and judgment that parts of our beloved Earth (home to billions of people) is evil, humanity can only respond by waking up to defend and protect Her. We, as humanity, the collective feminine and masculine, must respond with an opposite impulse, one of compassion, creating within our hearts an "Axis of Love" becoming ONE.

Is the Statue of Liberty not a splendid example of the Gaia leading us into a promising future? She recites! America the country in the West, becomes a haven for all. No not foreigners but the Light for future humanity.

> *Give me your tired, your poor,*
> *Your huddled masses yearning to breathe free,*
> *The wretched refuse of your teeming shore.*
> *Send these, the homeless, tempest-tossed to me.*
> *I lift my lamp beside the golden door!*

Being a Mother

In the expansion of infinite time and space, the human spirit **The One** incarnates on the Earth repeatedly in a process of evolving and purification to ultimately attain perfection. The choices of gender, female or male, are connected to the last gender oriented incarnation. If the pendulum of the male incarnation has swung too far out, meaning for instance that actions are male dominated and prove to be hurtful for himself or other human beings, the consequences for future visits to the Earth clearly must include an incarnation in which the roles are reversed and a vulnerable female life can be experienced.

By design the body of the human female carries the possibility to invite the incoming spirit present in the surrounding cosmos to spiral down into the deepest recesses of her body, the pelvis. In the human skeleton two distinct round bowl formations are found. One is the skull, which rounds off the height of the upright human being, and the other is the pelvis, which carries the weight of the internal organs. This roundness comes to perfection only in the female pelvis. We can create an image of this structure likening a Grail for the incoming cosmic spirit, the unborn child, **The One**.

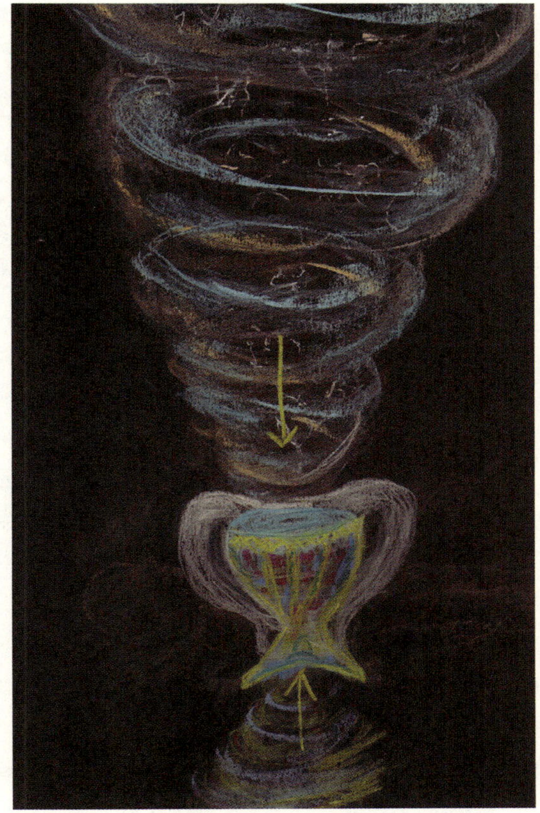

Plate 93: Female pelvis as Grail with double vortex

Not all female incarnations are given the opportunity to carry a child into the world and it stands to reason that I start to ask myself as a woman, how can such a task become a blessing or a curse. The young woman becomes conscious that every month again and again her reproductive system opens up to the invitation and fulfillment of a primary function of her body. Serious consideration must be given to the yearning, holding the small and vulnerable in her arms, to augment her loneliness with another being that she can call her own, or the desire to become an adult and find worth in the function of motherhood.

There are so many subjective reasons why a young female plans motherhood. Planning parenting without considering the incoming spirit being is irresponsible and therefore not acceptable. As parents we do not own the child, this means the child is not our possession, our play toy or an object to act out our own frustrations and desires. This being, **The One**, comes to the Earth to find the dignity of and protection for its own individuality. The ear of the mother is turned to the voice of the being that will come through her. She may hear or see it in a dream, months before conception. How many times have I heard the story that the child announced itself in urgent pleas to open the door for its entrance? It seems to me that even the father's role is delegated not as the parental donor but by the incoming ONE from a different dimension. Like lightning the conception can make an impact on the parents to be. Many parents can corroborate that the hour of conception was also for them very special. Through the pregnancy the woman experiences the wonder of a new life, the growth, the movement and the opportunity for silent but intimate conversations she holds with this new being.

Personally my pregnancy was one of the most authentic physical experiences of my life. I had embraced the idea since the age of fourteen. Being occupied with study and later an active professional life, not much time or inclination was spent on sexual matters. During my study in South Africa the male fellows assigned very little sexual appeal to the female students and this inferior profile continued to haunt me. One-and-a-half years before the conception, while still in the Netherlands, I had a dream. I was walking down the street of my childhood home, exactly the same place where as a five-year-old child I had experienced a clairaudient incident. There in front of me stood an old fashioned pram with the hood toward me. In a slow movement I looked around the hood and there was an adorable little boy, smilingly looking at me conveying a message: "Make haste; I need to come!" So how is an unmarried woman, not in a relationship and on the verge of immigrating to a new country, supposed to react to such a request? I realize now that "the word of God" even at that time was of great value to me. In my will I was obedient to an inner voice. Could I expect such decisive ruling from above, to have sensitivity for social mores of decency? In those years women were not supposed to act independently on issues of motherhood, and a child out of wedlock was not acceptable.

Yet I continued with the itinerary I had set out for myself and waited full of confidence for the next step. In time a revelation was imparted. The first year of residency in Internal Medicine was completed. America was great and I had fully acclimatized to the people, the work and customs. I had purchased a new car, was moving to an apartment in Brooklyn Heights, and anticipated a second year of residency in a large, well known Hospital. On the day of my first visit to the new hospital a few days before the work began, all physicians were invited to meet and introduce each other.

As clear as ever, even now, the following incident can be reconstructed. Through the door I walk, and in the front by the window a mature resident with a distinct accent, like we all had, explains the schedule. I observe him silently, somewhat confused with the many new impressions and the following statement I hear within " He will be the Father of your child!" This time I was overwhelmed mostly with disbelief, and the fact that again here I had no say or control over the situation. But mark my words this is how "it" works! The human being on the horizontal plane if it is in the service of higher beings will obey decisions, incomprehensible to our still-limited soul life. The only dialogue that ensued was a shoulder shrug later that evening, and the question "HOW?"

To make a long story short suffice it to say that this person, who was the head resident, serious and pious and exceedingly attractive, pursued me of all people. He was my type! In spite of the use of contraception, the entrance of "my" child was secured during our first contact. I now was assigned the role of motherhood without being conscious of the vast life changes that were set into motion.

All foreign students have to pass a flex-exam to obtain a medical license to open an independent practice in the States. The first opportunity to do so was in September of the second year of residency. It was a four-day multiple-choice ordeal and I had not done much preparation. What a surprise to receive passing results just one day after the discovery of my pregnancy! Now I could stay in this welcoming country, and secure a "home" for this new being. I had to fight for the unborn life, because the male partner was realistic in his evaluation that a pregnancy would be an enormous burden to him as well. Not wanting to demand from him, I felt strong enough to "do it alone."

No family, no intimate friends, my situation was a total secret. But of course there was help, and the decisions I made were clear and concise, and the steps taken toward the future were always an improvement from the present. I left the position as resident and moonlighted as an emergency room physician, which I could do with the license secured. I found a nice house to share in Astoria and the most lovely elderly couple to hover over me. I felt continually blessed.

My son, I knew it would be a male child, made every day of the pregnancy an unforgettable experience. On the day of the birth, my father was present, having made the long journey from South Africa. I fought for a natural childbirth, unheard of at that time. Breast-feeding, a natural instinctive way to succor the baby was not encouraged. For three days we lived a restrained existence in a separate hospital room. Once discharged, the care of the child stood in the center of my life and I could fulfill the role I had always dreamed of not expecting it would be granted. It is the being of the child I have to thank, for its willingness to enrich my life with such an opportunity. Such a thought may sound foreign to many, but the mood of this unconditional sharing, the emotional intimate caring the mother experiences, and the whole absorption with another being, enriches the feeling life for a lifetime. Of course many mothers go through this role but as the human evolves toward a consciousness it becomes more poignant and meaningful.

For me motherhood was an essential phase in my growth, a choice of the female incarnation that was totally in line with my destiny. Through the birthing process, I as woman learned to listen to the child's footprint on Earth. Through breast-feeding, I as woman experienced gratification in suckling and attending the innocent. Watching the first footsteps, I as a woman was reminded that the incoming being must establish independence. In attending to the child's development, I as woman must forfeit my own needs. It is inconceivable to most young parents that also the incoming being makes choices, choices of time and space, family connections and connections with old friends. I do encourage young parents to live for a moment with the image.

> The spirit of the incoming being soaring down on beams of light,
> created by the intimate love existing between the parents,
> to find a resting place in the deepest most secret part of the mother!

Of such a profundity is this image that it must have an impact on a female incarnation. Just turn to the child and say: "Thank You for choosing me, to teach me what selflessness is, to allow me the experience of unconditional love." As we embrace this being for a longer period of time, nurturing it and witnessing its footprints on Earth, the list of appreciation grows.

In the evolution of the human being the earthly incarnations are essential for the development into Divine beingness. The tasks assigned to me through motherhood often seem unsurmountable. There is pain because of plans and aspirations made for the child having gone astray. How can the mother embrace actions of a child that are not acceptable in a society? We can all agree that the burden of motherhood is one of the most far reaching and altering states in the life of a woman. It is the state of motherhood that is most exalted but also the most misunderstood.

Chosen by **The One** for its incarnation, it creates an intimate association between two human beings regardless of gender. Did it exist before? It surely will result in the continuation of a bond between two beings that is infinite and intimate on a soul-level. Especially the first son can become a light being for the Mother. This could become misconstrued as an overt bonding such as we can witness in dominating behavior of one person over the other. Pathological relationships become nurtured by insecurity and unhappiness of the unenlightened mother figure. Through the support of a strong family structure such situations can be recognized and prevented.

The Act of Marriage

The wedding feast is a celebration that draws people together in joy and communion throughout the world. As an institution it is sanctified before the community in a ceremony usual with a religious setting. It is legalized through the courts of law and gives the partners advocacy for each other regardless of the sexual orientation. The merging of Bride and Bridegroom as ONE stirs a deep-seated promise that the human being was not meant to be alone during its sojourn on Earth. Marriage must have a spiritual connotation, however the true meaning of this institution has eluded humanity. Contemplating the full meaning of the bond between two people, a bond so life affirming to entice also **The One** to merge, becomes a process beyond subjective experience. Monogamy is strictly a subjective choice for both partners in a sexual relationship not destined for reproductive purposes.

Why? The physical attraction between two persons is a spontaneous phenomenon, short lived and without a foundation build on trust. The pure lust and enjoyment for each other is born out of a self-centered need, and fulfills the purpose for that time. Freedom is maintained and no promises for future steps are considered. Discretion is a necessity for both partners involved.

In the medical therapeutic field it is recognized that a spontaneous orgasmic reflex is part of a physiological response mechanism. The sexual act for one or both partners can bring an orgasmic release. The act of onanism, though forbidden by the fundamental religious orders, is practiced with joy and dedication by both the sexes. In the last fifty years, pornography advertised and readily available through the Internet, has become a part of this cycle. It finds a fecund soil with the generation of those persons that have lost their own skills for a vivid imagination and become more and more addicted to the world of virtual reality. Explicit reenactments created by producers without scruples, who live in and through these sordid activities, remain lucrative and rewarding. In this world there is no room for subtleness. What you see is what you get!

The wedding, in contrast to the marriage, could be a joyous ceremony in a community, to recognize and support the intent of a couple in the interaction with each other on all levels. For older couples beyond the reproductive years, such a partnership is constructive, supportive, and will include care in the years of physical needs in the years of aging.

There is the reality, in the process of evolution, that embraces the concept of a "holy" partnership. More and more human beings will have a desire to start a "loving" partnership, with a like-minded person, who can be trusted and accepted and their totality even emulated. The practice of placing the other one before my own selfish tendencies becomes the challenge in such a bonding. The trust is necessary because both partners desire to live for, with and in each other. Such a liaison places the human child **The One**, on a pathway of maturation, embracing a potential for growth, and learning about the concept of unconditional love. Can anyone imagine what such a path would look like? Here two human beings, walking hand in hand, physically attracted to one another, in the process of dedicating their combined efforts to the growth of the other, weaving their destiny in a functional foundation to contribute to a society that protects them? The prerequisite of tuning in to the conversation of each other is known to me and the partner, I give space for the emotions of the other, my needs are clearly defined and I am in tune with the need of the other! Can you see that in this way a tapestry is woven, in which the threads of different colors are creating a unique cloth even a garment for a new entity or idea to join this small but powerful family?

The marriage becomes a necessity only for the protection of the incarnating spirit being. In the group of two a third party is invited and consciously allowed to enter. It is in the mood of desire from both the parents and a deep reverence for the procreation of a new earthly body that such a process can be initiated. The commitment to **The One** is as long as it takes for the young being to mature (twenty-one years).

Humanity learning about love is active in a process of evolving toward perfection. Studying the New Testament may bring me on a path of recognition that the protagonist, the figure of the baptized Jesus, was the Son of God. This supreme lofty being became the incarnation of LOVE. He is likened to the Bridegroom choosing as His partner collective humanity (the soul of humanity, *Gaya*) in its potential as Spirit Beings. In the future a wedding can be expected between the Bride (humanity) and the Bridegroom (the Christ-being) so that the metamorphosis into Godhood can be vouchsafed.

As Lover

There are invariable ways that I can move my love
It is not in what I do, but in being pure and spontaneous
An overflow of my deep love for his nearness,
his warmth and his ability to give so unconditionally.
I cannot fathom what goes in his mind, the power of his being,
And yet the little hesitation in his breath tells me
Of his complete captivation with something new to him.
The softness of his soul must frighten him
Out of control indeed he could get hurt.

But beloved, I give myself to you,
So that you can explore my being.
I need to be moved by you
Moved by your tenderness,
Eagerness to discover ever more
the variables you have kindled.
So it is the you and the me
Reaching out to touch
That which is Eternal
Love everlasting.

The Credo

For most people religious affiliations are kept private and somewhat obscure. To be associated professionally with an "evangelical organization" makes a statement not necessarily that "we are better" but an acknowledgment of a spiritual world (vertical plane) and creates a personal belief-system. Strangely enough for the disciples of Christianity, many twists and turns exists enabling also in this faith to have human opinions causing strife and dissent.

Stories of personal faith as much as our own bed or bathroom habits are so intimate that even with long-time friends, customs such as prayer, meditation, and reactions to subjective belief systems are often not questioned or revealed. Much was my amazement with a recent newspaper article wherein a "confession of faith" questionnaire was discussed. This poll concluded that in only the State of Mississippi more than sixty percent of the citizens were able to discuss their loyalty to their Christian conviction openly and with enthusiasm. This provoked my own questioning around authenticity and how the meaning of my life could be expressed as a unique testimony not of success but a continuous work in progress toward a moral imagination true to my personal "Confession of Faith."

The Apostolic Creed is recited by all members of the Community of Christ regardless of church affiliation. Most of this has become monotonous lip service that asks to be replaced by a bold individual conviction. As the conscious soul awakens in an evolutionary process of spiritual growth, the Self of the human being, **The One**, must be enabled, provoked so to say, to stand before humanity and state his or her conviction, "What I live by." Such an exercise may be difficult at a young age but it is interesting that the younger generation, being earmarked as the privileged aristocracy of Europe in the nineteenth century, mostly were encouraged to create such a Credo between the age of twenty-one and eight. Such Credos are found in historical contexts of (usually men) prominent persons who lead empires and civilizations, and are quoted in their biography. What are the considerations in fashioning such a document?

1) To be free of the influences of the learning institutions. The desire to test everything by experience.
2) To know out of certainty and inner conviction. Divine revelation exists. The perusals of the vertical plane.
3) To place a value of self within a social parameter. My place on the horizontal plane. Personal impact of my work.
4) Placing oneself in dimensions of time and space. Infinity.
5) Am I loved ? My desires in connection with this question. Can I experience Love?

The Credo emerges out of a human being in search of itself at a time in the biography when "I" starts to manifest (ages 21 to 28). The creation of such a document may be labeled as a totally selfish preoccupation, however one realizes at a later age, or the end of life; that revisions will be made once such a statement has been made as a conscious soul experience. The credo in a figurative sense has impenetrable boundaries around it and does not have to be shared with anyone.

Being a Doctor

In reviewing my life it becomes very clear that my destiny was intimately connected with the medical discipline and, as luck would have it, during the unfolding of my biography I was postured with one foot on the African continent where the witchdoctor, *tokolosi* still ruled in the rural areas of South Africa, and the other foot in the Western medical module, with an indoctrination into the materialistic mechanical scientific discipline that a natural science provides. In the end of the nineteen fifties the testing of knowledge was still done through oral conversation with our professors, and the written questions tested us on many levels of quantitative as well as qualitative scientific inquiries because our teachers still carried their own studies and interest into the curriculum.

Once I was situated as an independent voice in the role of a rural physician, it became clear that the threat of change hung over most physicians as the Sword of Damocles. The aspects of health care touted as essential to the future were listed as follows:

Legal persecutions from dissatisfied patients and their families; protect yourself (C.Y.O.A.) through high-cost insurance. With the increasing emergence of patient insurances, contracts were made between the insurance company and the healthcare provider, for whom an independent role as a physician was lacking. Group practices where as many as ten or more physicians signed up, were encouraged. The unique patient–doctor relationship was hereby endangered. Physicians preferred to become just a spoke in the wheel of the medical delivery system.

This was also the time that the pharmaceutical companies desired more power and decision making on treatment protocols. A subtle power play between the insurance companies and the pharmaceutical companies made it mandatory under the heading of "preventive medicine" to immunize all children and later the use of certain medication in patient groups of the practices the insurance companies had bought into. The reality was that Doctor-patient information was not confidential. Who had made these incisive decisions? Pencil pushers or the medical profession?

Diagnostic accuracy was delegated more and more to the diagnostic equipment the hospitals and group practices acquired. Once a diagnostic tool is installed for a very high price, all patients will undergo testing to defray the cost of the machine. I remember very clearly one wise colleague making exactly that point during a staff meeting of our local hospital, where the staff was consulted on the acquisition of a MRI machine at a cost of more than a million dollars. His insightful remark was, "Once the machine is installed, the patients will be lined up to undergo the procedure." These are some of the essentials contributing to the skyrocketing expenses of the bandwagon we call medical care.

During the years I practiced in this county, I was privileged to remain independent from all insurance companies, which guaranteed office confidentiality and a patient base whereby my patients would have to reimburse me for the time I spent with them during the consultation.

Arrows pierced my heart, so to say, with the realization that the future medical model would choose the mechanistic module. A practice in which the human spirit and life quality, dignity and personal biography are given attention was not recognized. For such an exchange, between the physician and the person who seeks advice (the patient) to take place, time and the willingness of the physician to be authentic and interested is necessary. As a physician I submit that all encounters will change me. I am molded, I transform, and I am used. How can these sacrifices be inculcated into the training of the younger generation?

This concept of healing as a living science in need of healers with a moral imagination is dying out, foreign in the Western education. Moral imagination as an individual strength is introduced here. This capacity requires young aspiring physicians to acquaint or be familiar with an inner silence, a resting of an overactive mind that is constantly reviewing. Herewith is enabled the enlivening of an imagination, drawing a picture of the patient with the Illness, to digest the pathology that is presented not only as a mechanical failure but taking into consideration the biography (thorough background) of the individual.

Does the solution come like a wind, immediately? Wisely we can say we sleep on it, and in the morning we remember that even at night we ourselves, as physicians, underwent a correction for the healing of the patient. I realize that as a physician I can heal nothing without the help of a qualitative entity related to unknown factors we can name Grace or the presence of the will to heal through me.

During the silence while practicing living imagination with the patient, thinking becomes an activity "it thinks in me." The method of healing is revealed—how to speak, what remedy to use, what test to order. The goal is to alleviate suffering. The soul function of reasoning, weighing opposites, and picturing the parameters of a living process evoke the activity of inspiration. This contributes to a conscious evaluation. A living thinking is here described. The medical discipline, extended by Spiritual Science, cannot be imagined in a culture steeped in natural science or in a materialistic worldview.

It is recognized that successful students present unique capacities, of which the most highly praised is memory, aggressive decisiveness, and mathematical thought processes. Individuals with strong idealistic "moral" values can barely compete with these demands. Personal attitudes have no place in the tutoring of the medical student who is exposed to the power of pharmaceutical manipulations and technical diagnostic advancements. The subjective becomes objective by teaching and indoctrination, following the laws of natural science. Expression of knowledge continues to be used on the horizontal materialistic plane in which time is finite and death is the ultimate demise of all life. Collectively, humanity welcomes a long life on Earth, abhors death and suffering, and rejects solitary existence. Natural science will continue to offer solutions to these impediments experienced in modern society. The curriculum of the medical study in the West concentrates on knowledge and memory of natural scientific facts, information that is reproducible and tested with multiple-choice questions. The Imagination of the student is stimulated through visual images on the screen. There is a threat that a Virtual reality could become the imagination of the future. Living thought processes, where the opinion of the student is challenged, is time-consuming and unpopular in many schools of higher learning.

We need to take into consideration that a fringe group of students of all ages are interested in the exploration of suprasensory phenomena and its resulting impact on human evolution. We still have freedom to investigate such research. Considering spiritual dimensions in the needs of our fellow human beings and developing the art of listening are essential tools in comprehending patients. If these discerning practitioners are discouraged in exploring the nature of the human in totality, a true healing will not evolve. A sturdy foothold in all future education must encompass the heritage of a reincarnating entity, the commonalities the human being has with nature and cosmos, and the knowing that there is more to life then only the horizontal. Natural Science must be augmented with a Science of the spirit. If squelched we negatively influence our own return to a future life of freedom.

As physician, with the experience of fifty years as an active practitioner, the intrepid dangers of the medical module we now are dealing with must be recognized. By needs, the modalities of diagnostic tools, pharmaceutical intervention, and mechanical surgical corrections have become the pillars in triage and are guidelines in adequate equalized care for all. If something is wrong with the body, "we" will correct it! Continuation of these practices obfuscates the role of the "healer." In modern medical care most physicians can forgo the title, the honor, the respect, the distinction, the role of savior, and so on, as long as they are paid commiserate to the title, a salary that is astoundingly high. Gradually, the distinguishing title "doctor" will be usurped, too, because the desire exists for ultimate control by a few people. Was it not proven that the heartfelt intimate role of a "healer" as a person who emerges from the university with a medical degree is not necessary?

Medicine is an art as long as it remains recognized as such. In the Germanic-speaking countries to receive a medical degree makes a statement that "I become a practitioner in the ART of medicine." This does not carry a title "doctor." That title should be earned through rigorous university training and a thesis after earning a master's degree. This title "doctor" would indicate an educational leadership to those pupils coming after.

To practice the art of medicine and healing I take into consideration that I can also resort to what I know from my own being-ness. It is authentic, individualized, a reflection of my own "thinking about" and the urge to experience a subjective solution to "healing of the other." When a piece of art is placed in a museum, people come to view it because it radiates beauty, is uplifting to the viewer; in other words it radiates an healing power. When the patient and the physician sit together searching for a solution to the imbalance claimed as an illness, unseen powers flowing from both persons and family, play a role in the exchange. A time element is introduced in the interaction. It takes time and an intimate environment for a process of enlightened exchange to occur. The visit to the "doctor" must reflect a quality of listening, silence, and compassion. It becomes possible that the circle of such an exchange widens to encompass many impulses or beings. Insight into "the other" comes from sources of inspiration and intuition. In truth, the physician can never claim the "healing." Modesty and integrity become second nature to the healer. The exemplary life of an alchemist is emulated. It was the alchemist who could still claim, "Change and be changed!"

Requesting a chair in a Medical college named "Life Philosophy" would be new. We recognize this in Hermes Trismegistus. Not wanting to reinvent the wheel his postulates are still valid and will in the future create the scaffolding for truth and accuracy in healing. It is not modest to make claims about the efficacy of the art in medicine extended by Anthroposophy. After all in this practice I advocate that the patient precipitates the healing process and as a physician I am the guide. However no guide can make progress unless a map is available, a scaffolding that provides a clear picture of a person with a genetic profile, incorporation of time and space in his biography, an evaluation of the resilience of etheric forces, the effect of the astral organization on mobility and mental stability and last but not least the recognition of the individuality that shimmers beyond all the discoveries like the light of the Sun illuminates our life path. What the true individuality can identify with its aim in this earthly life must be recognized and supported. That becomes healing.

Far from giving advice, guidelines for each of the hundreds of patients sitting down with me have been beneficial. I am willing to share these with practitioners of future generations, young people who have submitted to the shrinking process of scientific methods, endured night and days without respite and have survived that process. The generation before us must lead the way through their desires, dreams, creative urges, and hear the voices of encouragement.

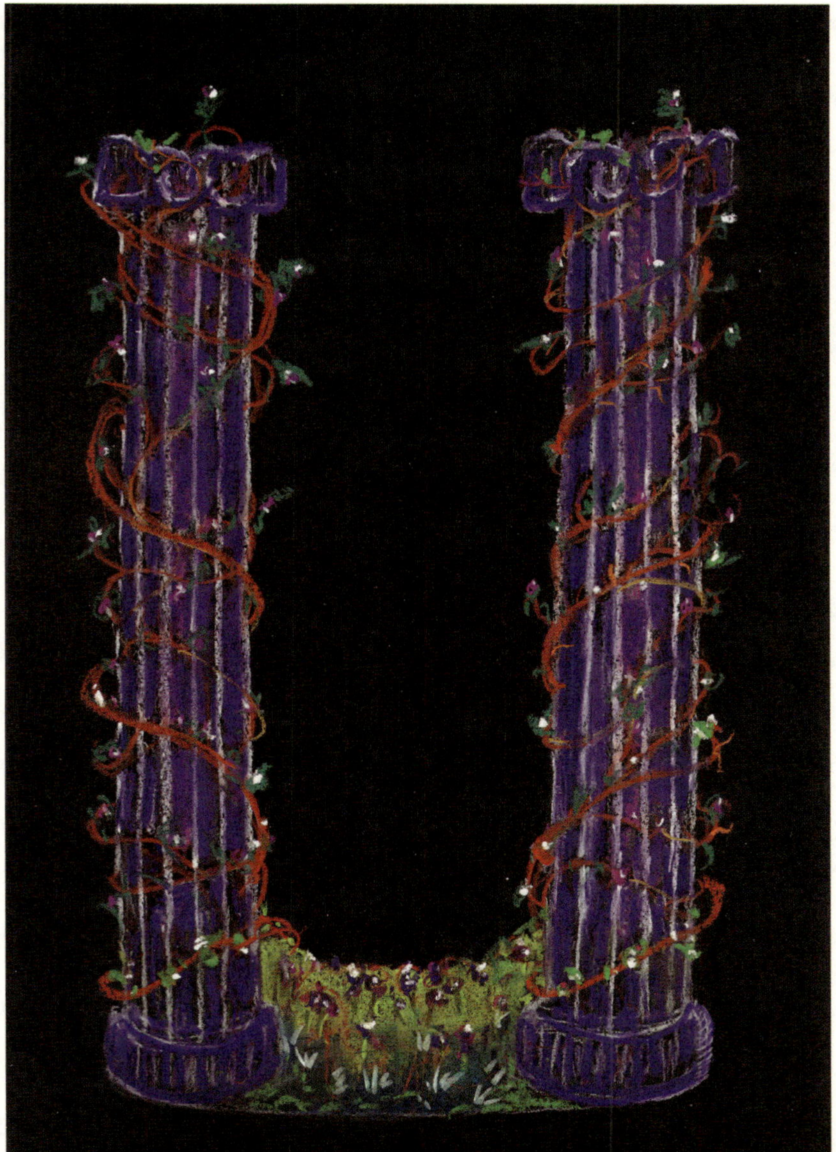

Plate 94: Sound U as depiction

Sound U

Unique, Universe, Ubiquitous, Utopia, Eulogy—all words beginning with the strong U sound, indicating or reflecting wholeness, an ideal being fulfilled. In the U experience I arrive at the conclusion of my life. This becomes the experience in where I stand like a pillar securing the human structure I support. Rooted steadfast in the Earth, upright, I reach out beyond the skull, arms covering the ears, high straight in a parallel formation touching realms of heaven. Who am I? Who is waiting? What will the future bring?

Subjectively, the U section of my life very much is reflected in the heavenly music of *Das Lied von der Erde* composed by Gustav Mahler. As the music of the last stanza fades softly, I find myself in full consciousness on a threshold of a new beginning stretching to infinite distances. Listen!

> I stand here waiting for my friend;
> I wait for him to take a last farewell.
> Where are you? You have left me alone so long!
> Oh beauty! O world, drunk forever with love and life!
> Where am I going? I shall wander in the mountains,
> I am seeking rest for my lonely heart.
> Still is my heart, it is awaiting its hour!
> Everywhere the lovely earth blossoms forth in spring and
>   grows green
> Anew! Everywhere forever, horizons are blue and bright!
> For ever and ever.
>
> —**Gustav Mahler**

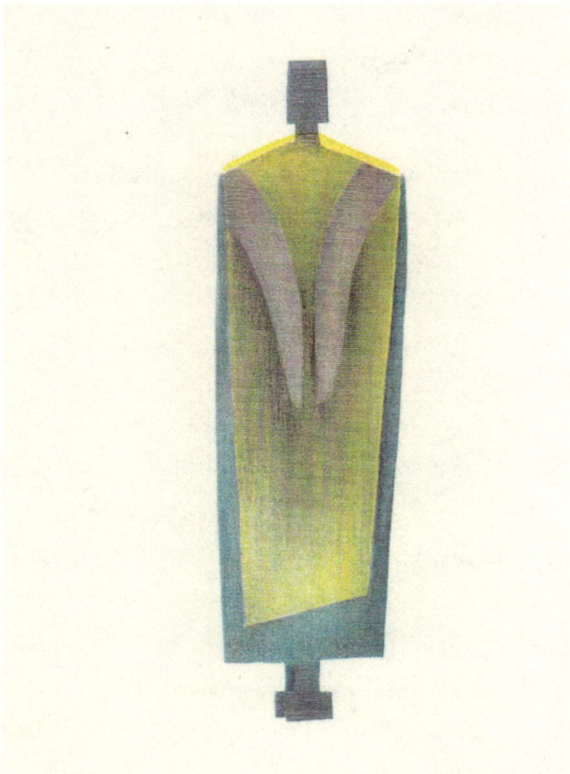

Plate 95: Eurythmy gesture of U

It is the last song, dedicated to the poignant farewell of the Earth-dweller. I am filled with the heaviness of parting, the yearning for the loveliness of Earth's infinite cycle, birth and death and the unknown dimensions of the future. Where will I go?

In contemplating my review of what is in the past, understanding the life of my contemporaries has value. Future goodness is born in us from our accumulation of past life experiences, now leavened by the yeast of wisdom. What was not considered before beckons with a tantalizing urgency. Writing, poetry, music, reading, research, are all explorations for which time is made available. Could one have hoped for such enrichment later in life, meeting aspects of the self totally foreign if not given the time to contemplate?

This section is dedicated to the review and further illustration of all the ideas that were introduced throughout the book. A repeated question concerns the fourfold organization of the human and the request for examples. I can find these layers of activity reflected in the historic stories collective humanity carries throughout times immemorial, the myth, fairytale, fable, parable, and legend.

The myth would be connected with the physical accomplishment of a person, an outstanding feat that would memorialize such a man or woman. I am reminded of Joan of Arc who in a female body accomplished such a remarkable masculine task. The myth remains hidden to us until we reach a stage of physical independence.

As children we are privy to a wealth of fairytales, stories that rise out of the collective unconscious, stories rich in symbolism, stories that are imbibed and require no explanation. These tales fall under the heading of creations arising out of the life force present in all of humanity, stories connected to the ether body as a commonality in us all.

The fable and parable become familiar to us later in our development when as human beings with a consciousness we can say: I stand corrected, My Bad! The emotional ripening depends on the astral body and fully occupies our beingness after sexual maturation.

It is only in the legend that the individual "I" begins to weave the tapestry its own identity on Earth. The threads can have the quality "I" choose, varying between luster and dull gray. The feat of individualism we can only reflect upon after the biography is completed. An authentic review of such a life creates the legend.

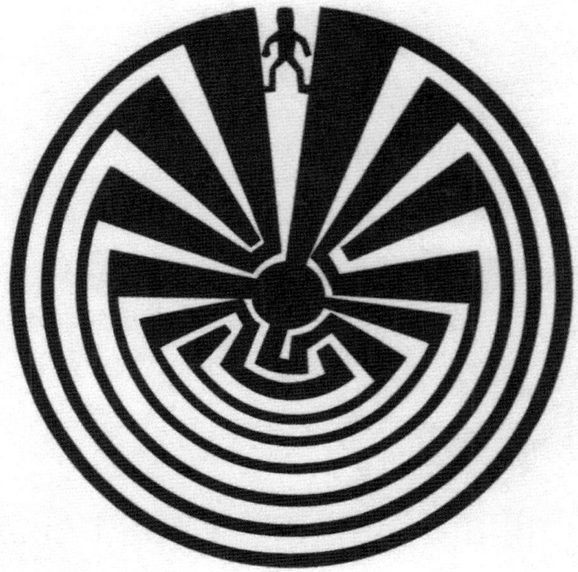

Plate 96: Life becomes a walk through a labyrinth

In the evolution of humanity the stories become reflections of soul as is experienced on Earth in the past and present. As the human is still a "work in progress," future stories will be written that reflect the evolving godliness of humankind. What stories would those be? Of sacrifice, reconciliation, and triumphs? Humanity will always accumulate and present stories. Intimate, personal, authentic reflections of life's laments and triumphs enrich the traveler during its sojourn on Earth. In the art of storytelling and representation of the images, all of us find solace, hope, and Soul.

The Physical Organization, Myth, and the Vertical Plane

Each person when born, owns a unique physical identity, be it a footprint or DNA, to make a claim on being a part of the human family. Birth becomes a weighty proposition when we examine the physical body in the light of such an individual representation. With or through the existence of the physical body on Earth, heroic deeds will be remembered in story, song, and pictures. As the time goes by, the biography as a story takes on a mythical quality. As we learned from **The One** finding its "home," deploying its boundaries at the moment before conception, the opportunity for a preview is extended. Still protected by the "arm of the angel," choices in gender and genetic disposition (all physical accouterments) will be chosen while the blueprint of its personal myth is viewed. The question lingers: "In which physical garment can the earthly task best be accomplished?"

Consider the assignment given to Joan of Arc (1412–1431) also referred to as The Maid of Orleans. At the age of 18 she played a heroic role ending the hundred-year conflict between England

and France with the Siege of Orleans and subsequent victories for the French King Charles II. Yet this individual chooses a female gender, within a peasant family. Only the Angels could foresee the appropriateness of such choices.

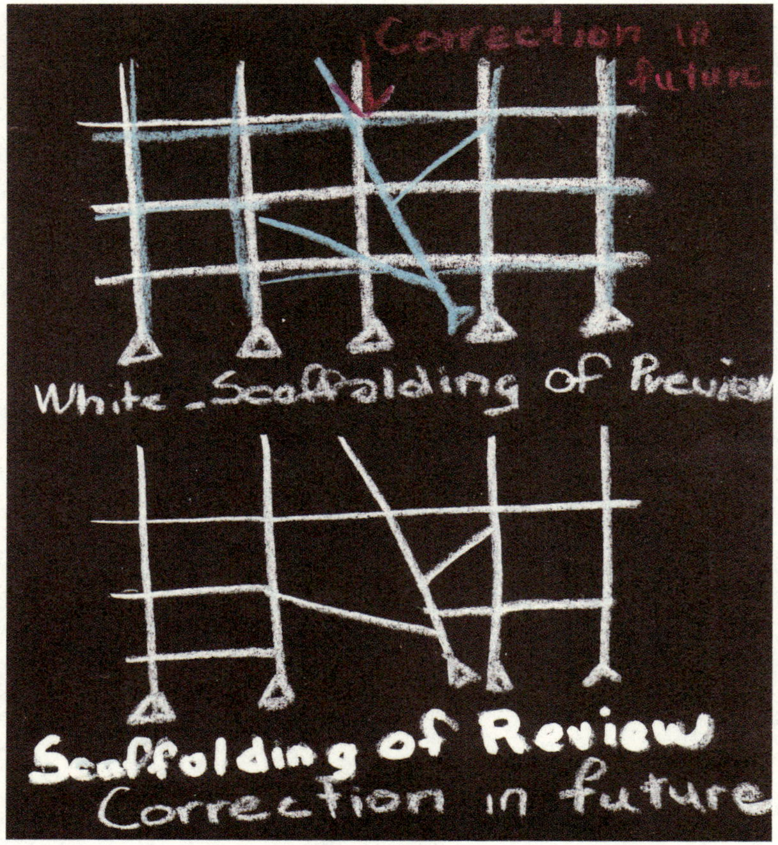

Plate 97: Preview and review

In fulfilling its Myth, **The One** takes into consideration the task for the immediate future, its life on Earth, and the connection with its assignment needed for such an accomplishment. The preview although hidden in the recesses of our unconscious, will again be examined in the process of departure from Earth. The review of life is experienced with our last breath (the near-death experience discussed in section on immortality). The availability of both suprasensory views becomes like two blueprints that will be displayed for comparison once the physical body is left behind. There are beautiful images available in museums in where the Egyptian Pharaohs after death had to face the trial of weighing the heart for purity of thought and intentionality of the will. In the beginning of our life a burning desire to accomplish is experienced and at the end of life a consternation to find that the blueprints do not coincide. Where have we gone astray? Where did we take a wrong turn? The discrepancy between these two blueprints, the preview and the review, becomes a contributing source for the material accumulated for further review of time spent between two earthly lives. "To do it better the next time" is the sincere hopeful greeting the Cherokee exchanges on the departure from this world.

The text in all the sections remind the reader that throughout **The One's** life there is a deep knowing that an higher order avails itself for its protection, guidance, and accomplishment of ideals. Most people are oblivious to these admonitions and even with a religious background, give scant validity to spirit also experienced as the Higher Self. The plane of the vertical dimension, a plane where higher powers are recognized, a plane in which **The One** can discover its interaction with "the beloved," must become accessible to all. For we as human beings are mostly striving for worldly goods and fail to review our day with the question: "Are we still on track with our ideals and fervent desires?"

How can I share with the reader the experience of preview and review as a contribution to the imagination? Can such experiences happen randomly and anywhere? An experience as this is placed outside of the senses, but can become a percept on account of memory. Not involving the outer senses, one becomes immersed in pictures, voices and even scenery that are multi-layered. In our dream-life such images are created and with training waking recall can develop. Playing itself out, beyond the physical body, the perceiving organ is not of or in the body and must be recognized not being bound to one dimension—vision, for instance. With hearing we experience sound all around. The vertical plane surrounds the probing quiet investigator, and will reward it with spontaneous insights. We can call them inspirations and intuitions. The observer imprints the supra-sensory stimuli as memories. Unexplainable, they are yet experiences that must be real.

Using the physical body will allow **The One** to contemplate the marvel of its atomic structure and the lawfulness of its natural chemistry, reveling in a superior and unique upright structure while moving on Earth. The capacities beyond these gifts enables **The One** to prepare the mythical story of heroism, to reconnect the bridge between two worlds and to dedicate itself to the evolution of the species. Most of the time however, introducing, reviewing, and evaluating the story that each person lives by on his or her earthly walk can only be done at the moment of death. We can hear many such stories during funerals of our family members, friends, or acquaintances, but mostly the lines of the eulogy are often confabulated and not authentic.

What of course needs to develop is the capacity to listen to the inner voice in oneself. No story can unfold with noise around or in you. With an imagination your own myth becomes authentic and manifests throughout your life with a stubborn certainty. The story continues. The development of a personal confession of faith, also referred to as The Credo, is an exercise for the individual after the age of twenty-one. This becomes a final concrete testimony of the "I." Contemplating your own essence, not what people around you want, but what it is you can give, is the foundation of growth and worth.

Etheric Organization and Fairytales

Beginning with "Once upon a time" and ending with the phrase "and they lived happily ever after!" wraps the child within all of us in a blanket of security. Over and over these anecdotes are repeated, and curiously enough each child has his or her favorite. This collective material still alive in the unconscious folk soul all over the world hardly requires images through fancy books, movies, and theme parks. Suffice it to assume that the content speaks to and satisfies the child on an unconscious level carried from generation to generation. I would even suggest that the creation of explicit virtual realities such as have been introduced in the Western culture exploits the child's imagination and therefore damages. The stories of witchcraft, of suprasensory beings in nature conversing with the protagonist, family members that act out of malice or evil intent are definitely palatable to most children and play a role in their fantasy. It is still a world of make-believe. However a deeper connection to the functional body systems may be detected because the enactment of these stories becomes therapeutic. The question arises. Can we find a fruitful Imagination between these collective stories and our bodily functions? We find it in the four organs, each one with their distinct function and contribution to chemical constitution. The etheric body contains within its parameters of forces four distinct characteristics identified as *fire* (warmth), *light* (air), *tone* (water), and *chemistry* (minerals).

I can find definite connections with the fairytales left to us by the Grimm Brothers in stories connected with the formative forces of the organs, warmth ether, light ether, tone ether, and chemical (or life) ether. These living stories had their origin in tight communities where elders received recognition for their "knowing" and were sought after for their wisdom. The lay person had an ear, could understand the stories woven by the older people of the community, stories weaving on a deep unconscious level into their own healing powers. The last phrase confirmed the resolution and success story.

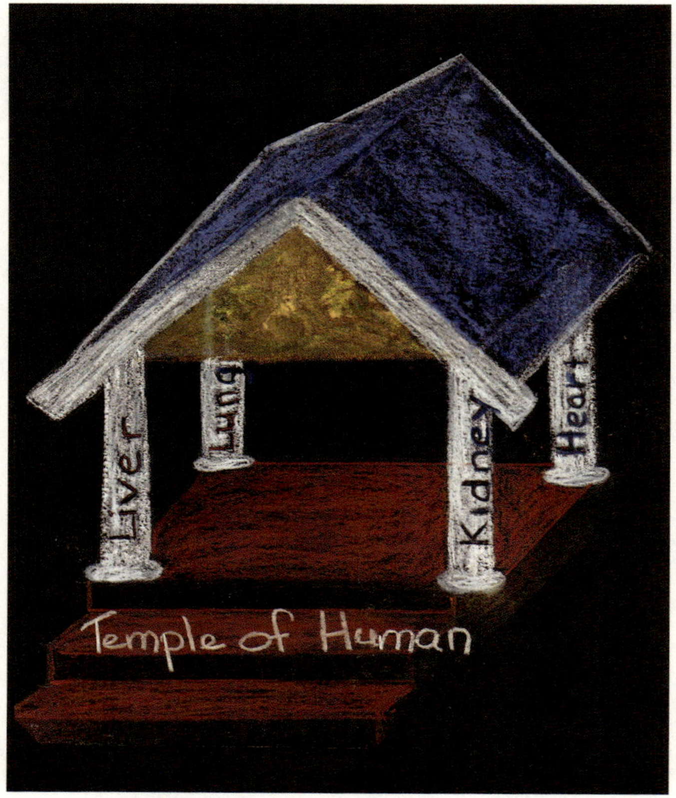

Plate 98: Temple with four pillars

Ending with the phrase "They lived happily ever after!" the listener, usually a child, collected the images before sleep, digested them at night, and healed the wayward stalker within its own unbalanced body. Healing does not necessarily indicate a return to balance but certainly a shift from a deep hidden nature to gainful insight into the pathology so that it can be worked on in the day-consciousness.

The content of fairytales can direct the "organizer" of health, the etheric body, to bring balance where there is an abundance or shortage of the warmth, light, tone or chemistry, to "set things right" in the natural function of the body. Only then can the cells in their distinctive function "live [together] happily ever after." The body as an accumulation of different cells can in this sense be interpreted as a living entity interacting together for the health and balance of the whole.

Let me introduce the wide variety of organ function, as the seed material for your own story. In our daily life nothing is as personal as the habits we display over and over again. What are my Habits? My bodily organization carries deep from the interior involuntary movements, facial tics, and the way I move, laugh, speak, and convey myself to the world. Habits, acquired on Earth are well nigh impossible to change; they are so to say the signatures of who I am and are a part of the etheric organization.

Like four pillars carrying a roof of a Greek temple, the four organs of our physical body—the kidney, liver, lung. and heart—fulfill a task by conveying a personal profile. Is there a link between the four organs and the habitual gestures we incorporate? Through acquaintance with the other person, whether close family, friend, or neighbor, I can identify a distinct signature in each person. On the physical level what becomes unique is the DNA, a combination of thousands of protein building blocks also named the amino acids. Such a spiral shaped protein becomes the foothold for the formative forces special within each one of us. Individual proteins present in the body fluids are a component of the "living water" we previously described. The etheric body sometimes is referred to as the *habit body*. The Physical body carries the distinct chemical make-up of the DNA. The etheric body contributes to the unique habitual profile of the person.

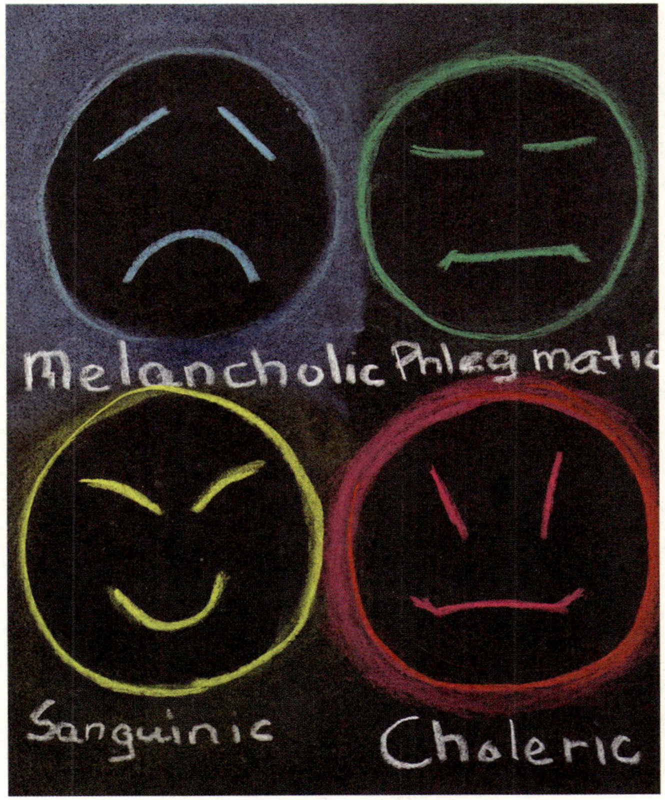

Plate 99: Facial gestures

The Liver

The four organs are a source of our habitual life. Let me explain this with the following Tale that is connected with the Liver and Gallbladder organs. The story familiar to us runs as follows:

Prometheus, presented to humanity as a son of Zeus, visited the Earth frequently and sympathized with the laborious life humanity had to endure. Then being sleepy and experiencing no fun, he endeavored to bring in the arts of music, dance, weaving of colorful cloths so that their lifestyles could be enhanced. For this Prometheus was punished, being that early awakening of the sentient soul life was against the wishes of the ruling god. For forty long years he was chained on the rocks of the Caucasus Mountains, day and night, and only the Eagle devouring his liver starting at sunrise, alternating with sleep at sunset healing the wound over the night were his companions. This circadian rhythm of the liver was hereby introduced with the bile excretion commencing at sunrise, approximately four a.m. for twelve hours, followed by a liver metabolism for the next twelve hours. This circadian rhythm has become habitual for the etheric organization connected to the liver/bile organ. A constitutional weakness in the liver gallbladder system that usually can be diagnosed would cause a disturbance in these functions and open the door for pathology.

Habitual profile is not only reflected in the presentation of the body (*gestalt*), but also the emotional reactions of that person. On an emotional level, the liver gallbladder synchronicity has a far-reaching influence on our temperaments. Are you a choleric, full of fire? Your bile is strong and the temper is close to the surface. In the case of a melancholic, one's bile is black, sticky, and slow moving. This person drags through life with a heavy mood, downcast and negative. For the sanguine personality on the other hand, life is a blast, dancing, scurrying, with many places to visit but with a short attention span. The phlegmatic typifies the balanced organized methodical liver type, trustworthy, steady like clockwork. We know for ourselves that temperaments cannot change. The etheric signature stays with you in this life until the end of days!

The liver system is designated by the two diametrically opposed physiological functions of construction and excretion. These can be imagined as a polarity. With the one pole responsible for the anabolism. (A constructive process by which a cell takes from the blood the substance required for repair and growth, building it in to a cytoplasm thus converting a non-living material in to the living cytoplasm of the cell, typically storing energy.) The other pole, catabolism (excretion), includes all the processes in which complex substances are converted into simpler substances, usually with the release of energy and excretion.

Anabolism	Chemical/Life	Endothermic	Centripetal	Liver
Catabolism	Warmth/Light	Exothermic	Centrifugal	Bile

We can wonder if here also the etheric organization with its four distinct formative forces of warmth ether, light ether, chemical ether, and life ether is not functionally designated, to each of the metabolic opposed region. The liver organ itself dominates the centripetal chemical ether and life ether forces, those forces that function as gatherers of substances, and give form to living water and chyle. The bile in the ducts and the gall bladder, display the centrifugal activity of the warmth ether and the light ether, with outward radiation, heightened activity influencing transmuting chemicals into waste products in a process of catabolism.

Out of the interplay between polar opposites your personal story, the fairytale unfolds. The liver being such a mighty organ gives shape to the personality, the fluctuation between moods of abundance or frugality mentally designated *mania* and *depression*. The fairytale itself often uses a gender distinction between the two lead protagonists, for instance the bewitched sleeping princess and the traveling, courageous rescuing prince, opposite actors or forces finding balance through each other.

In mental disorders, one can certainly attribute bipolar disorder to a liver constitution that runs in families, therefore of a genetic disposition. Here an imagination that one of the pillars of the temple (which is our body) is not able to carry the full load of function on its "shoulders." From this information can I assign the reader to create a personal profile? Does the repetitive push and pull of these organs find an expression in my own habitual presentation in life? Give self-examination a try. Can you recognize yourself in your liver function? Do you have a liver profile?

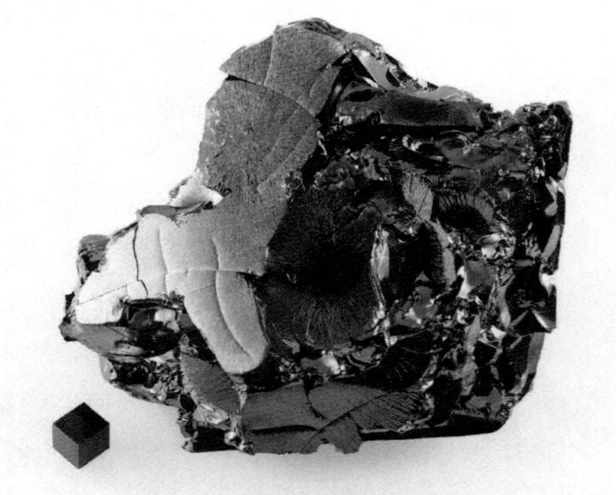

Plate 100: Carbon

The Lung

The lung organ, for its transmission of life-giving air into the blood, has a different tale to tell.

Let's not look objectively from the outside at the ribcage that so perfectly protects the lung and heart. Imagine crawling inside and having a subjective experience of the constrictive feeling of imprisonment behind the horizontal bars of the ribs. It becomes elementary that the exchange between inhaled Oxygen and exhaled carbon dioxide involves the entrapment of Oxygen molecule, by a Carbon molecule associated with all life on Earth.

Listen to its riddle,

I am an Atom with greedy hands
Reaching out to many a friend
Holding on to all my brothers
Become pitch black like the others
Crushed by the heaviest of weight
Will then release the purest of light
In the Kingdom of plants I will provide
Skeleton, structure and scaffold aside
On Earth I make friend in flower and fruit
Fashioning colors and patterns for suits
I marry many a bride but am loyal to none
Dancing with water gives all a spin
Bedding with nitrogen I sentence to death
Merging with Oxygen gives new breath
Like a bird in the sky. I rise and set free
Life on Earth I have to flee
I organize nature, order abounds
For the created One chained to the ground
I release and set free to return to beyond.

If I am asking myself what substance defines the Earth, the answer can be found in this versatile Carbon molecule. Our planet, solid earth is constituted out of a mixture of silica, aluminum, and carbon. However an alien visitor would find an abundance of the carbon molecule throughout all solid substances, water, and air and come to the conclusion that on this planet the carbon molecule is an indication of life forms existing from the beginning, because Carbon is connected to life or the living kingdoms as we know them.

The lung organ is utilized to bring the Carbon of the air to the small alveoli and here it becomes active in the mechanism of exchange of all the solid substances suspended in the living water of the physical body. Through inhaling, Oxygen is supplied to the blood and the excess of Carbon is exhaled. The breathing mechanism is totally unconscious in a steady seesaw motion: In—Out—In—Out... A weakness in the organ of the chest cage affects my breathing so that suddenly I become aware of an arrhythmic function. I heave, I pant, I sense hunger of air, I suffocate, and I am imprisoned. Like the bird in a cage I become restricted in my movement, I am unfree, I have to submit to a reality of being locked up with a bag over my head. Despondency overcomes me because I and the solidity of the Earth have become one (Grimms' fairytale, *Joringel and Jorinda*).

One can have a mental experience of restraint if constitutionally a genetic weak lung "pillar" is diagnosed. Daily I can be confronted by anxieties that hinder me in the free expression of myself. Questions like, "Have I turned off the water?" "Is the door locked?" Also in an obsessive profile, with phobias and compulsive tendencies, I can recognize myself not being free, in other words, I am a **lung** personality. These personality traits are strongly dominant through family lines and therefore have a genetic disposition. It becomes a challenge when these personality characteristics can be interpreted with a fairytale innuendo. What story could I fashion for myself and how could my tale end in "Living happily ever after?"

Notice that the feminine and masculine aspects are both present in the fairytale. Carl Jung (introduced in the section on immortality) unraveled the significance of his personal psyche as a gender duality he then referred to as *animus* and *anima*. Did he stumble on the life activity of the formative force within himself? Did he not find in the male who in his sexual organ is bound by the centrifugal formative forces of warmth ether and light ether, the urge to vanquish, dominate and possess? Then, the same free radiating formative forces present in the head pole now, as his muse, a feminine companion, his Beatrice (a soul in Dante's *Divine Comedy*). The opposite picture can be constructed in the psyche of the female, where she experiences body-bound compulsion to receive the domination, water clogged, indolent, and slow to escape, she rather submits out of her nature! Her triumph comes in the form of the prince, in shining armor, riding a white fiery steed.

Aah! These are the fantasies with which our psyche rescues us from a life of doldrums! They are symbols of people, animals, and fairies, all part of the collective memories of humanity and hidden as the formative forces of each organ. One functions in life out of the formative forces that are unique to each one of us. This organization penetrates the solid, earthly body (the ashes). With my "death," these forces will be released into the cosmos, becoming a part of the collective memory of the world.

The Kidney

The Kidney as an organ of excretion has again a different story. The expression "Urine is the mummy of the astral body" was left to me by my mentor in medicine extended by Anthroposophy Otto Wolf, MD, a master in the art of teaching and storytelling. Leaving his pupils with such a statement guaranteed our continuous loyalty and dedication to the (as of yet) unknown riddles the living body presented. This section is not intended to concentrate on the astral body but to look at the kidney not only as the organ for excretion but to search for the anabolic as well as the catabolic function—the polarity. Urine consists of dead water (ninety-five percent) and solids (five percent), the latter being in a solution. The kidney acts to maintain homeostasis of the blood and body fluids. Physiologically, the renal system can be divided into two contrasting functions. It is certain that the anatomical kidney has to submit to a constant vigilance, each drop of blood is scrutinized by a glomerular body that looks like an eye. Why? So that I can see you better, smell you better, taste you better! (Little Red Riding Hood). That contains the story of this organ, an inner sense organ.

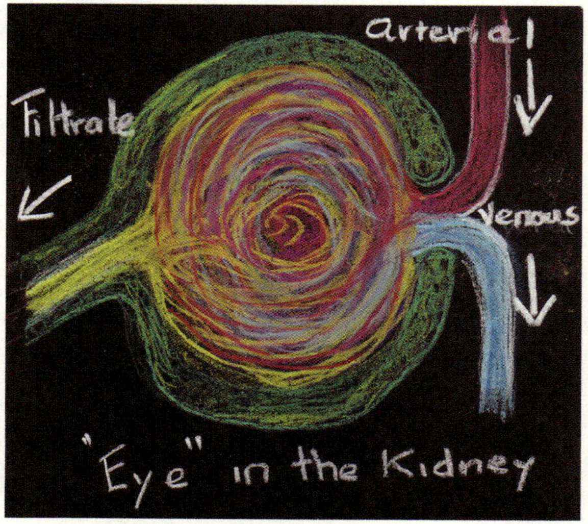

Plate 101: Malpighi body

The anabolic function of the kidney is connected to transforming and maintenance of living water. The catabolic function results in the excretion of urine (dead water, the mummy). What is living water? This fluid body occupies ninety percent of total body weight. It cannot be compared to urine, blood serum, or a synthetic liquid in which all the constituents of organic and inorganic molecules are dissolved to imitate body fluid. Understanding the concept of "life" we enter the world of an imponderable quality, the etheric organization. This becomes a realm where I have to divert my thinking from the non-living concept, to incorporate the living cell in its reality. This cell has the capacity to stabilize itself constantly, thanks to the etheric life force present in all living. This would mean that ninety percent of our physical organism is assigned to the task of maintaining the life function. It penetrates the whole bodily structure sleeping or waking, and has anabolic and catabolic aspects that are self-regulating.

From the renal system the living water radiates toward the entire organization. Living water permeated by the etheric organism moves toward the entire organism. The etheric organism is completely permeated by imaginations. This is important to know if I want to make a story of my own organization. The imaginations are pictures of my own organism. For my consciousness to be activated in these images, stimuli from the exterior senses and my conscious brain activity have to be pushed to the background. In a dimmed state such as in sleep, or focused meditation we can enter a world of inner self-perception, a world of rich imaginations reflecting for instance the anabolic metabolism during sleep. These occasionally rise up into my consciousness as dreams or pictures with hidden symbolic connotations. In this state we meet our dreams.

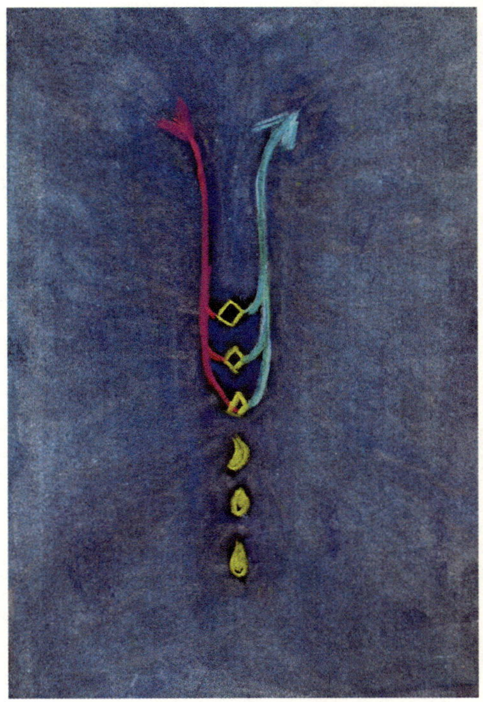

Plate 102: Imagination of living water

Through the removal of substances from the blood through the process of filtration and selective reabsorption, the toxic catabolic discards of especially protein metabolism are dissolved in dead water and excreted. The excretion of dead water, which contains the end products of metabolism, helps to regulate the water, electrolyte, and acid base content of the blood.

As we can gather out of the previous discussion, the kidney organization in its expression of its formative force be it warmth ether, light ether, chemical ether or life ether, supplies the person with a rich imagination that can feed a vivid picture for the collective unconscious. Any condition that loosens the adhesive quality between the physical–etheric bonds, conjures subjective phenomena that on the mental level are named schizoid. Cannabis and LSD are known for their hallucinatory quality when ingested. The weakened physical–etheric bonding causes flashbacks. This causes free flowing warmth ether or light ether to circulate and penetrate the consciousness. Here the brain functions as the mirror to the imaginative pictures carried in the etheric organization of the blood.

Kidney radiation can be extremely unpleasant, and are in many instances a reason for

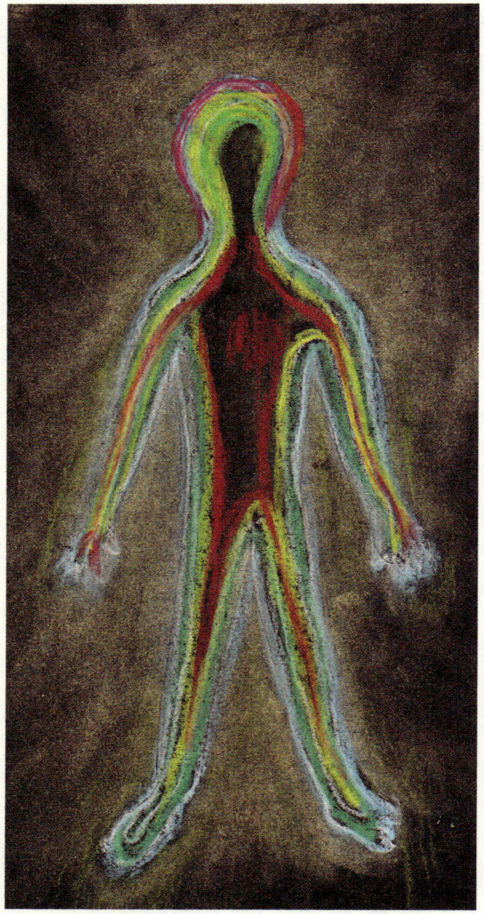

Plate 103: Bonding between physical and etheric

mental breakdowns and consequently hospitalizations. On the other hand the kidney personality can lead us into a world of rich images. Books most children have enjoyed and read voluntarily, emerge from the unconscious weaving of a kidney personality who can analyze and use the rich imagery streaming from the interior to enrich all of us (J. K. Rowling, the Harry Potter series).

Completing the four organs responsible for the construction of all amino-acids in the human being, the scaffolding used by the etheric body is the basic formula constituted of Carbon, Oxygen, Hydrogen and Nitrogen (COHN), with multiple permutations thereof. I use an imagination of the substances named atoms and molecules, circulating in the blood coming from the digestive nutritional stream (chyle). The molecular formations are enhanced by each of the four organs through the specific activity of the living water from that organ (being etherized). As a result, an utterly unique protein is enlivened in which the mark of the DNA makes it decisively personal.

The Heart

Lastly we examine The Heart, which adds Hydrogen to the formula. We can reflect on the previous organs with

earth—lung/Carbon
water—liver/Oxygen
air—kidney/Nitrogen
fire—heart/Hydrogen

I feel in myself the order of nature in these fourfold structures and as an earthling a certain satisfaction is derived out of an exact progression. Can the heart be called an organ? On the physical level processes of anabolism and catabolism are not identified. The heart is not a pump, it can only be called an organ of propulsion. Branco Furst (*The Heart and Circulation*) points out the essence of the heart function to be more like a hydraulic ram, which is set into motion by the constant pulsation of the peripheral flow of blood to the center. The heart is built out of muscle tissue, damage to this muscle by vascular impediment or a traumatic contusion results in diminished heart action. Adequate blood flow to the muscle is the hallmark for any healthy active muscle.

The arterial, capillary, and venous parts are integral in the blood-organ circulation. Movement of the blood originates out of the periphery and streams via the venous system back to the heart, seen as the center of the circulation. However I have learned to accept that for true pump action, the heart muscle is not capable. One could feel sorry for the heart because of its continuous muscle activity, but if we watch a picture of the electric impulses streaming between contractions it is evident that the heart of all muscles chooses its activity judiciously and wisely. Temporally the contraction (systole) occupies one third of the period (beat) where the remaining time is spend in a mode of restoration (diastole). Good for the heart!

And do I have a story? Well the heart does not have a story. It is a story! This story is witnessed in many modern languages as expressed in the synonyms with which we express the purity, courage, warmth, honesty, openness, compassion, tenderness, caring, and sharing of friend and neighbor in our community. The hidden capacity of the heart becomes an experience to the other person, the quality of which is objective. The radiating quality of the heart forces is carried and expressed by the bearer as a light that shines in the dark; it personifies the beauty of humanity, the certainty that evil can be overcome, and the hope for a light-filled future. On all levels the story of the heart will become the story of humankind, the more we are encouraged to adhere to "My Imitation of Christ" (ref. Thomas à Kempis).

In Latin the word *cor* is used for the heart, and it is amazing at how many modern European words contain this small, three-letter word to express the quality of might and power. Language carries the intimate desires to express those emotions we all want to share.

Have the courage of the Lion when exploring your heart's desire.

The Astral Organization: The Parable

The sequence of events in the life of Christ after the christening by John the Baptist in the River Jordan has been told by many of his disciples as well as biographers in the last few centuries. We are not privy to conversations with the friends close to him. What is remarkable is that most of His teachings were conveyed for posterity in the form of a parable from which the reader or listener could extract a message that was meaningful to their own life situation. The prerequisite for such a teaching meant that the receiver was attuned to his own emotional needs, awake to the needs of others, and equipped to discern the vices and virtues with which all humanity would have to deal in earthly life. The institutions of religion thrived on the interpretation of these parables, and for nearly two thousand years desired to think for the "sinning" human being. All personal stories that are made by humans are for the humans, and emerge out of that part of the human being we designate as the astral body. It is easily remembered that the astral body derives its name from the moving and the fixed stars. Certainly the astrological observations by the priests in the Babylonian Civilization (3000 BC) contributed to the wealth of imaginations that guided humanity's emotional evolution from the primitive aggressive homo sapiens to the more subtle, civilized, emotionally controlled individuals who were learning to live in harmony and peace with each other regardless of background.

However, that humanity needs to be reminded over and over again that we must continue to live by guidelines, that each vice has a virtue and vice versa, and that personal effort in control of emotions becomes the hallmark of maturity, designates all members of humanity as a "work in progress." We are here in need of further exploration. How can emotional maturity be advanced through our own volition and knowledge?

The heavens spoke to the Babylonian astrologers thousands of years ago, in the "language" of the living moving world of the animal kingdom. For them it was natural to think of the human being as the center of the universe, **The One**, and that vertical existence is reflected in the planets and the zodiac. Those priests were the namers, and their laws remain valid today.

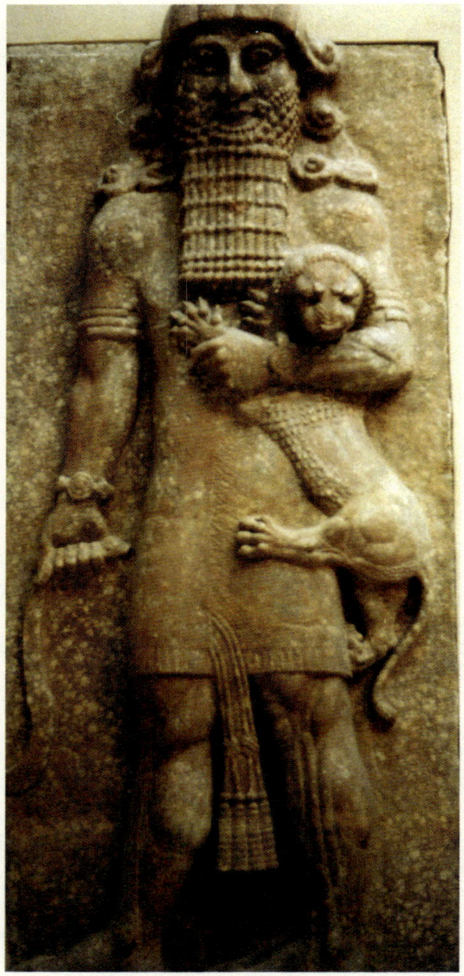

Plate 104: Enkido embracing the lion

Here are some of the laws that have been carried over into modern star knowledge: Both the moving stars (planets of our solar system) and the fixed stars (members of the zodiacal belt) influence the human being. The body of knowledge associated with this discipline is called *astrology*. Different signs of the zodiac and the planets are dominant at the moment of birth for every person and connote a specific signature.

The heavens make a complete circle around the human being in a twenty-four-hour time frame in one day. The belt of the zodiac is divided into twelve regions, most of them reflecting the signature of an animal. Twelve-month division is earmarked by the calendar months we use in a worldwide timely order. The fixed stars move slowly around the Earth in a circle of 365 days. One year. The New Year starts at spring equinox on March 21. This is not a date used as a significant calendar reminder.

At the moment of birth the configuration of the heavens is imprinted in the etheric organization of the child. (It is possible that the configuration starts already at the moment of incarnation of **The One** during conception. (Refer here to the work of Willi Sucher. *No new research on such calculations is forthcoming.*). For the female child born with a fixed amount of ova, the Sun–Moon angle at birth will determine her ovulatory cycle at the start of reproduction. The Sun–Moon angle will indicate the time of ovulation.

With careful study and observation of animal habits one can frequently notice parallels in the human. The similarity between human profiles and the animal world is a source for humor but can often help us in an evaluation of the peculiarities in our fellow citizens. It is also true that humans living on a farm often take on the characteristics of the animals they care for.

The student of the animal kingdom understands nature's wisdom and how a complete assimilation of the animal in the wild allows it to survive hardships. It is the humanization of the animal that makes its survival precarious. The need for closer bonding to the animals has become a curious phenomenon in Western civilization where the members of the animal kingdom, especially our pets are submitted to human standards.

Cruelty to animals is punishable. An animal in its nature is cruel, but obviously emotional trauma is at a minimum. The capacity for reason in the soul of the animal is absent. When a human being behaves "like an animal" we meet actions that are despicable, and it is mostly assumed that as a human being "We should know better!"

The animal astral body is uncomplicated and rests in its genetic inheritance. In contrast the astral body of the human, although animal-like in the scaffolding, can be modified, molded through cultivation, and carries responsibility for its reactions in the world.

The human is placed on the Earth to care for his fellow human beings. The opposite reaction occurs, creating a climate of war and destruction caused by the overwhelming fact that for each human being born the first thought is of the self. The inherent nature of all human beings is centered on the self. It follows that the human being acts instinctively out of its own insights. Freed from the domination of nature's imprint, thinking, feeling, and will (soul activity) replace this restrictive role of nature and, reaching beyond the animal imprint, create a distinct human activity in which self-thought dominates. Where the animal is not capable of violating the natural law and order, on the other hand, the human being oversteps natural laws continually. Examples are,:

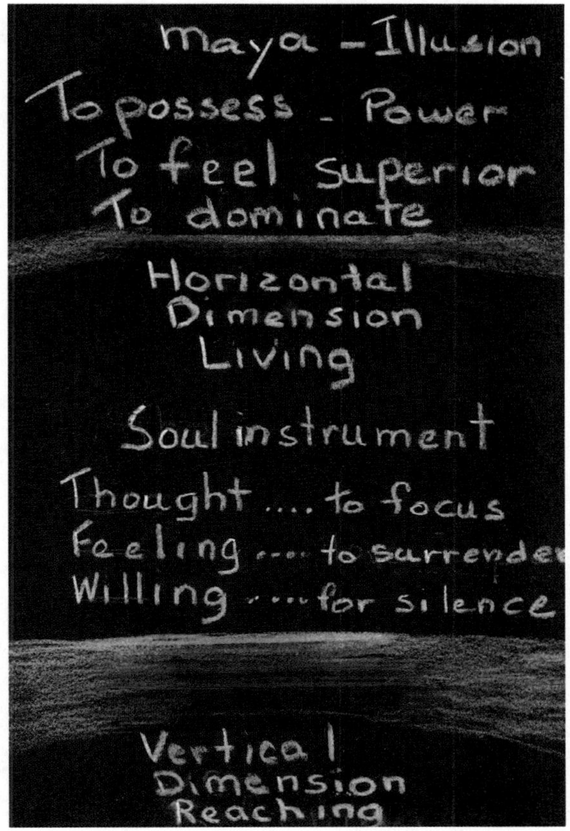

Plate 105: Maya—illusion

1. Overlooking the world-truths wherein all people are equal. Through seductive and misguided thoughts the appointed leaders of nations are encouraged by their followers to destroy "inferior" factions of humankind. Superiority as a qualitative or quantitative evaluation can only be used in the material world, the dead world. The living world gives us the challenge to respect the dignity of life.

2. Harboring false and sentimental emotions; the illusion of power and dominance and the willingness to submit to such ideas at the cost of losing our freedom (relinquishing our human freedom to the idea of world power).

3. Belief that the mechanical driven world will triumph. In such a world the idea of brother-/sisterhood will be obsolete. Slowly the wisdom inherent in nature will be ignored (destruction of life-sustaining fauna and flora for financial gains and dismissal of the small for the big)

Equality, Freedom, and Fraternity were the cornerstones in the French Revolution and subsequently continued as ideas in the New World when the Constitution was written.

Conflicts and dysfunction between persons in private life as well as the working place arise out of the array of vices donated to us by the celestial hierarchies. Self-interest dominates; consequently, these vices become challenges, and when consciously emoted, become the configuration of the personal astral body.

There are twelve vices we can identify and are associated with the zodiacal segments that are present in a 360-degree circumference around us throughout the year (Paul Platt, *The Quality of Time*). This researcher dedicated long years in personal observations regarding the reign of these celestial segments on our astral body and the emotional effects one can observe during waking time (refer to plate 80, page 75).

The best defense against negative emotional patterns is the knowledge of one's own human nature or personality. Giving attention to identifying the animal profile within oneself, and learning about the astral patterns and emotions that go unheeded will bring insight and clarification. Such tools are necessary for the transformation in character, a growth needed in the process of maturing (F. Julius, *The Imagery of the Zodiac*).

Children learn from the fable through identification with each protagonist. The story often ends with an admonition encouraging the child to become conscious of the plight of the underling, the trodden, and the hurt. "The moral of the Story is. . . ." Moral standards are introduced, with the recognition that the human can have choices that are unavailable to the animal.

The astral organization plays its role in the dimension of time (days, months, and years). The rotation of the Earth as planetary body, places the human being under a continuously varying experience of cosmic forces throughout the year. To explore these qualities of time with our own inquisitive mind is the hallmark of the human being. Remarkable is that every minute of waking consciousness an infusion of negative feelings bombards the astral body and in reality no one is free of such an onslaught.

What one learns when observing one's own comfort or discomfort, the emotions one experiences during confrontations with the world, the reactions manifested in meeting new circumstances, all become colors on the pallet used for painting the biographical tableau. Emotions and reactions become the conscious experience of virtues or vices. We can thank the creative Gods for bestowing these hurdles on humanity. What comes toward me in this incarnation will determine the path I choose to walk.

As long as the will exists to change, the signs of the Zodiac holding the secrets of the vice, has been one of the best foundations for understanding how to approach areas of personal uncertainties, to bolster self-worth, and to overcome hurdles in human interactions. Rigidity and separation from " the other" must be resolved to make room for accessibility, affinity, and affability.

The "I" Organization: The Legend

It is at the end of a life that the world traveler will pose the question: "What will I be remembered by?" In the Eulogy a review of the memories will inform family, friends, and colleagues of the endearing, brave, and outstanding qualities of a beloved person. There is sadness around the impending separation. But the eulogy is not the legend of the person. Such a story only unfolds in a time long after the individuality's sojourn on Earth, giving the individual time for the review after separating from earthly reality.

The Legend has a pure individual expression, and I imagine it to become the garment for the Being in its next existence on a different

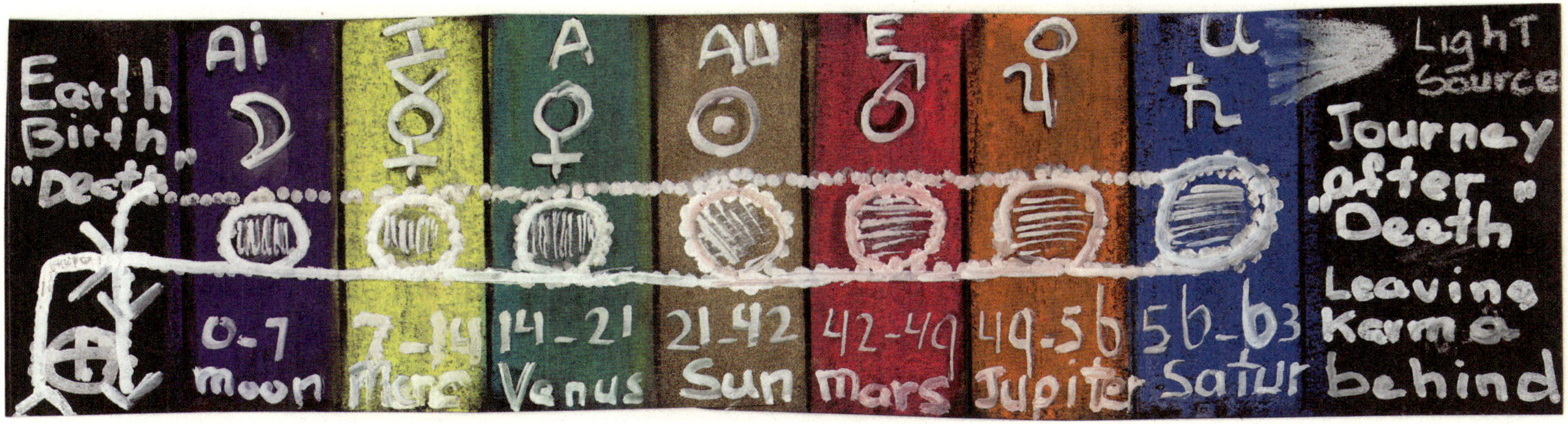

Plate 106: Leaving karma behind

plane, in a new dimension. I do not know the legend that will adorn me in future existence. My Legend is an unknown entity, unless it may be connected to the Credo I was able to fashion during my contemplations on Earth. It seems to me that it becomes important that I was understood as individuality. Have I made myself clear? Was I able to express the confession of my personal convictions in my daily activity? If I had a shimmering of my higher self, could this be conveyed to other humans? I was able to write down the requirements for writing a credo, rules of faith I live by, in the previous section. This alone becomes an urgent invitation for **The One** during its daily routine to consistently examine motivations, followed by the question: Are my actions authentic? Am I true to my intentions?

In the act of living, daily gathering is continuous. This action is from periphery to the center. We all will face a birth in a new existence. To equip ourselves with a garment of truth, beauty, and goodness becomes a goal for our earthly life. Those are the contributions with which we will enter this new existence. What will be the garment?

I bring here a final story of transition witnessed in one of my patients. On his deathbed, there came a defining moment when he threw of his covers, slipped out of his bed, stood erect holding on to the table for stability and with one last breath expressed in a loud voice: "I want to be free!" At that moment his transition became a reality, he excarnated! While leaving the realm of Earth, the horizontal plane, he was fully conscious and able to step eagerly into another existence, without any fear or uncertainties. Was this his legend?

Once we can leave the restrictive earthly body, a journey through our universe can be undertaken and can be expressed in terms of an expansion. Orderly is the progression, following a similar path as to the travel on Earth during sleep every seven years, further and higher. The spheres of Moon, Mercury, Venus, Sun, Mars, Jupiter, and Saturn are all visited and are represented as ever-increasing intensity of light and illumination. I imagine that the hierarchies in these celestial spheres are occupied with nothing else but to expand the understanding of the individual, an understanding of functions and form connected with the physical body. This becomes the knowing with which The One will return to repeat the cycle and reconnect with the beloved *Sophia–Gaya*.

My daily life is occupied with the thoughts about the past, the present and the future. People I was destined to meet, the changes I have witnessed, specifically the deleterious effects on the youth, has spurred me on to impart my concerns and apprehension of what may help for the future. In this way I hope to contribute to a process of curiosity and awakening **The One** in the reader.

Epilogue

Knowledge of my existence as infinite, is a reality given to me through grace at such a young age that it was not shared nor questioned. As my life unfolded many encounters, memories, and stories with other human beings have accumulated, which give birth to this testimony of **The One** weaving the intricate pattern of destiny on our planet Earth.

The introduction of a belief system was unacceptable and I had no need to adhere to doctrines most of which thrived on sentiments of superiority. The concept of "belief" created uncertainties in all decisions I had to make. On the other hand a "knowing" deep within my heart provided me with an empowerment for the daily activity throughout my life.

All that I learned from studies was not only memorized but integrated into a scaffolding of realities and became acceptable truths. I followed a voice within, nudging me to differentiate between "the tree and the woods." The question as to who spoke with an unassailable guiding voice within me became the leading motive for an investigation into suprasensory realities, the acquisition of which I assigned to a vertical plane. The curiosity for such knowledge continued to accompany me throughout my studies and in the life journey I was privileged to undertake. It was curious that in the seven-year stages of my life new certainties emerged from the "sea of unknowing" to enrich the horizontal life I was living beyond the mundane.

Only after the age of forty-two my continuous enquiry around a dominating figure mentioned in stories of evolution throughout the world, was answered and solidified in my own mind. Testimony of a visitation to our planet by an Avatar needed to be explored.

The writings of Édouard Schuré (*The Initiates*) and Rudolf Steiner (The Gospel of St. John) illuminated the path toward the certainty that Christ as a fiery alien light-being, who claimed a human body, walked the Earth for three years, left a body of teachings transmitted through the Bible, and remained deeply connected with humankind. This became a new overarching reality in my life. Sentiments of infinite allegiance and the riddle as to how to validate such a discovery in day consciousness stirred my daily activity.

This life-shaking conversion ripened over a seven-year period, finalizing in the realization that opposing forces, destructive, seductive, and evil did exist, continually luring **The One** away from possibilities of spontaneous allegiances to the God-spark in all of us. I heeded the voice reminding me that the lonely path of individual action needed to be recognized.

Yes, I now experienced being alone but never lonely. The voice accompanied me throughout time and space. I trusted it, obeyed the suggestions that were sometimes scary, and found succor in the knowing of the unswerving fidelity and love for me.

My practice shifted from a conventional method of internal medicine in which quantitative evaluations were encouraged. Pursuing a quality in the consulting hour demanded that all members of a family were introduced. I was repeatedly challenged to practice a medical art that was extended by wisdom of the human being in its truthful representation of an evolving body, soul, and spirit. The new patient entering this sphere of healing made often a conscious choice to work toward a self-recovery and demanded to be in control of its own healing process.

Such an interaction opened new worlds to me, introduced ideas of support in the impulse of self-healing, and acquainted me with age-old philosophies and knowledge the modern medical student was not privy to.

The tenacious execution of methods in healing I had been unfamiliar with up to this time, required trust, self-reliance, and enormous courage. Developing my own spiritual discipline and creating a pathway for the "help from above" was a mandate in this process of growth.

What I came to realize was that a Christianized medicine began with each of my patients, the moment it was recognized that the empowerment for healing was inherent in him or herself.

The individual is a work in progress. A mechanical medical intervention interferes with self-healing. Being sick calls for introspection by the patient eventually guided by the "healer." In this process support from finely diluted substances (homeopathy) derived from nature facilitate restoration of the balance needed.

The One is not alone. The four kingdoms it experiences on the horizontal plane surround it. From the celestial spheres it receives continual support in the thought forms of constructive guidance and affection. This world speaks in me; I will be introduced to it only if I give room to hearing the voice. Our mandate is to listen. A path of understanding will lead to freedom.

The introduction of the Child Artist in my life and the work that was prepared by him for all of humanity was a voice of the modern human searching. On an unconscious level he was persistent not to let his message slip into nothingness. To do so meant a sacrificial act, experiencing hell through the path of substance abuse and poison.

The human interaction between the "healer" and the "patient" is continually interchanging. We end up with the question: "who heals?" This is answered with a certainty that each human being becomes the medicine for and remedy of the "other."

Could this fact prepare us for a future where compassion as a spontaneous function of the heart will develop?

See me
Feel me
Touch me
Heal me...
(The Who, *Tommy*)

References and Recommended Reading

Alexander, Eben. *Proof of Heaven: A Neurosurgeon's Journey into the Afterlife.* New York: Simon and Schuster, 2012.

Anonymous, *Meditations on the Tarot: A Journey into Christian Hermeticism.* New York: Tarcher, 2002.

Aristotle (384–322 BC), *Internet Encyclopedia of Philosophy* (http://www.iep.utm.edu/aristotl).

Appenzeller, Kaspar. *Die Genesis im Lichte der menschilichen Embryonalentwicklung.* Basel: Zbinden, 1989.

Blechschmidt, Erich. *The Beginnings of Human Life.* New York: Springer, 1977.

Cockren, A. *History of Alchemy* (http://alchemylab.com /history_of_alchemy.htm).

Dunselman, Ron. *In Place of the Self: How Drugs Work.* Stroud, UK: Hawthorn, 1993.

Emerson, Ralph Waldo. *Essays: First and Second Series.* New York: Harper Perennial, 1951.

Erasmy, Hedwig, MD. *Cosmic and Human Evolution.* Chestnut Ridge, NY: Mercury, 2003.

Fischel, Alfred. *Grundriss der Entwicklung des Menschen.* Berlin: Springer, 1937.

Frieling, Rudolf. *Christianity and Reincarnation.* Edinburgh: Floris Books, 2015.

Furst, Branko, MD. *The Heart and Circulation: An Integrative Model.* New York: Springer, 2014.

Jocelyn, Berendene. *Citizens of the Cosmos: Life's Unfolding from Conception through Death to Rebirth.* Great Barrington, MA: SteinerBooks, 2009.

Julius, Frits H. *The Imagery of the Zodiac.* Edinburgh: Floris Books, 1993.

Kempis, Thomas Á. *My Imitation of Christ.* Brooklyn, NY: Confraternity of the Precious Blood, 2014.

König, Karl, MD. *Embryology and World Evolution,* Freiburg: Verlag Die Kommenden, 2000.

Lauterwasser, Alexander. *Water Sound Images: The Creative Music of the Universe.* Encinitas, CA: MACROmedia, 2007.

Maintier, Serge (ed. R. Patzlaff). *Speech—Invisible Creation in the Air: Vortices and the Enigma of Speech Sounds.* Great Barrington, MA: SteinerBooks, 2016 (see also Johanna Zinke).

McGraw, Jamie. "The life and Legacy of Hermes Trismegistus." *Alchemy Journal,* vol. 3, no. 4, 2002.

Mead, G. R. S. *Pistis Sophia: A Gnostic Gospel.* Blauvelt, NY: Garber, 1984.

Nahm, Michael. *Wenn die Dunkelheit ein Ende findet: Terminale Geistesklarheit und andere ungewöhnliche Phänomene in Todesnähe.* Amerang, Germany: Crotona, 2012.

National Institutes of Health. "Stem Cell Basics," https://stemcells.nih.gov/info/basics/1.htm (verified 2016).

O'Neil, George, and Gisela O'Neil. *The Human Life.* Chestnut Ridge, NY: Mercury Press, 1990.

Platt, Paul. *The Quality of Time.* Self-published, 1982.

Rittelmeyer, Friedrich. *Reincarnation: Philosophy, Religion, Ethics.* Edinburgh: Floris, 1990.

Roob, Alexander. *Alchemy and Mysticism.* Berlin: Taschen, 2014.

Schuré, Édouard. *The Great initiates*: A Study of the Secret History of Religions. Great Barrington, MA: SteinerBooks, 1989.

Schwaller de Lubicz, RA. *The Temple of Man,* Rochester, VT: Inner Traditions, 1977.

Steiner, Rudolf. *Eurythmy as Visible Speech.* London: Rudolf Steiner Press, 1984.

———. *The Gospel of St. John.* Hudson, NY: Anthroposophic Press, 1984.

———. *How to Know Higher Worlds: A Modern Path of Initiation.* Hudson, NY: Anthroposophic Press, 1994.

———. *Intuitive Thinking as a Spiritual Path: A Philosophy of Freedom.* Hudson, NY: Anthroposophic Press, 1995.

———. *Man and the World of Stars: The Spiritual Communion of Mankind.* New York: Anthroposophic Press, 1982.

———. *An Outline of Esoteric Science.* Hudson, NY: Anthroposophic Press, 1997.

———.*Theosophy: An Introduction to the Spiritual Processes in Human Life and in the Cosmos.* Hudson, NY: Anthroposophic Press, 1994.

———. *The Wisdom of Man, The Wisdom of the Soul, and the Wisdom of the Spirit* (out of print); new edition: *A Psychology of Body, Soul, and Spirit: Anthroposophy, Psychosophy, Pneumatosophy.* Hudson, NY: Anthroposophic Press, 1999.

Stolp, Hans. "Het wonder van terminale helderheid." *Verwachting,* no. 74, 2015 (http://www .stichtingdeheraut.nl/).

Van der Bie, Guus, MD. *Embryology: Early Development from a Phenomenological Point of View.* Driebergen, The Netherlands: Louis Bolk, 2001.

van der Post, Laurens. *Jung and the Story of Our Time.* New York: Vintage, 1977.

Weihs, Thomas J. *Embryogenesis in Myth and Science.* Edinburgh: Floris Books, 2012.

Weldon, Laura Grace. "Mother and Child Are Linked at the Cellular Level." http://lauragraceweldon .com/2012/06/12/mother-child-are-linked-at -the-cellular-level/ (2012).

Wikipedia. http://en.wikipedia.org/wiki/Alchemy.

———. http://en.wikipedia.org/wiki/Gundeshapur.

———. http://en.wikipedia.org/wiki/Hermes_Trismegistus.

Wolff, Otto, MD. *De Mens in zyn Chemisme,* Studenten Werkgroep Geneeskunde en Anthroposophie, n.d.

———. *Grundlagen einer geisteswissenschaftlich erweiterten Biochemie.* Stuttgart: Verlag Freies Geistesleben, 2013.

Zinke, Johanna. *Luftlautformen.* Gerabronn, Germany: Hohenloher Druck, 1978. (see Serge Maintier).

Acknowledgments

The autobiography of a professional woman in a new country is studded with meetings positive as well as negative. All encounters have contributed to the embroidery of my own life journey and molding.

My first friend, Diana, initially a buddy on the ski slope, soon came to share her family, home, and table in spontaneous gestures of hospitality so typical of the old Italian roots present in our community. The warm embrace of welcome seemed to be most prominent with those folks who counted as immigrants from the Mediterranean regions as their forefathers. Eddy and Cathy Stiffler became friends, neighbors, and confidants throughout the time of acquiring the farm and beyond. Without Craig Schools' filiality toward the animals on our farm, my expression as a farmer would not have been possible. The folks who always stood by my side include Leah, Joanna, Judy, Joyce, and Melissa. I cannot imagine being without their enduring patience and loyalty.

My writings and impressions on life have been formed by the review of my peers and friends whose input I appreciate. Outstanding meetings I value and appreciate with the younger generations that have come before me. Starting in the 1960s, the incarnating souls reflected an astounding evolution. They showed interest, curiosity, and an iron will to complete the task they set out to do. My son Peter Pupator is one of them, and I feel profound gratitude for his dedication also to the material that was really a part of my story. Alex Schneider, always willing to give jovial contributions, brought me through the times of despondency with my inadequate control of the computer screen. All these, my younger friends Michael, Stacey, Heidi, Andrew, and Arthur, I have understood, and they in return have lightened my way.

Encouragement to make my own blackboard drawings, where possible, came from a wonderful artist herself, Sylvia Hough. She especially captured the moods of the texts, and her contributions beautify this testimony. I thank her for plates 27, 29, 30, 37, 39, 40, 48, 72, 74, 83, and 94.

The generation born in the nineties contributed in a new way. These young and often prominent incarnated souls did not ask for personal attention. Being able to carry them in my consciousness awakened in me the eagerness to share the results of the maze in which my life unfolded. Certainly the Child Artist gave me a reward by sharing his artistic story in spite of his own struggle to find meaning in his life. This generation has something to say, and they remind us to listen.

List of Plates

1. Standing boy 1
2. Signature as symbol 2
3. House, tree, person 3
4. The Hierophant 4
5. Metamorphosis of hierophant to house 5
6. Comparative drawing of home 6
7. Alchemical Oven 6
8. The Green Truck 7
9. The Devouring Monster 8
10. Process of consolidation 9
11a. Drop formation—pelican eggs 10
11b. Drop formation—sickle 10
12. Departure from Sun region 11
13. Cosmic sled in choppy waters 12
14. On Earth—end of journey 13
15. Temfor embryogenesis 14
16a. The Rudder (fragment a) 15
16b. The Rudder (fragment b) 15
16c. The Rudder—headpiece of the hierophant 15
17a. Dispersion—artesian 16
17b. Dispersion—fountain 16
18. Gesture of consolidation 17
19. Consolidation—embryo 17
20a. Heart (fragment) 17
20b. Flower (fragment) 17
21. The initiation of kings 18
22. Sun (fragment) 19
23. Symbols in the Sun 20
24. Face of the Moon 20
25. Tabula smaragdina (Latin text) 21
26. Sophia photographic imprint 23
27. Infinite heritage 25
28. Horizontal versus vertical planes of reality 26
29. Equilibrium of two poles establishes health 27
30. Plant as upside down human 28
31. Triangle and additional dimension 28
32. Fourfold permeating body 29
33. Space for vowel sounds 31
34. Horizontal time element of speech 33
35. Vertical space element of speech 33
36. The seven life processes 34
37. Sound A as depiction 34, 35
38. Eurythmy gesture of A 36
39. Distraction 37
40. Focus 38
41. Snowflake 40
42. Cumulus cloud 40
43. Salt mercury sulfur process 41
44. Archetype human form 42
45. Three Kings (reproduced) 44
46. Reproduction of Green Truck as comparison to alchemical equipment 45
47. Return of the Devouring Monster 46
48. Sound E as depiction 47
49. Eurythmy gesture of E 48
50. Image of Sophia 49
51. Soul genesis 50
52. NASA nebula 51
53. Heart (reproduced) 54
54. Cosmic sled on choppy waters (reproduced) 55
55. The Guardian (fragment) 56
56. Contributions of three beings 56
57. Gender chromosomes 57
58. Incarnation of The One. two activities and its completion 57
59. Fertilization 58
60. Dynamic attraction 58
61. Buddha. above as below 59
62. Morula 59
63. Depictions of the homunculus 60
64. The journey 60
65. Body stalk carrying three layers 61
66. Child Artist's depiction of embryo (fragment) 62
67. Embryonic developed fetus tucked in womb 64
68. Vowels in air 64
69. Cymatics in fluid 65
70. Hierarchies of Earth 66
71. Process of invagination 67
72. Sound I as depiction 71
73. Eurythmy gesture of I 72
74. Discover soul activity 73
75. Two sisters 74
76. Sphinx 75
77. Journey of "I" in sleep (0–21 years) 76
78. God Mercury with winged feet 77
79. Sleep and separation of astral body and "I" 82
80. Zodiac belt around the fetus 83
81. Birthday 88
83. Granny's grave 89
83. Sound O as depiction 91
84. Eurythmy gesture of O 92
85. Soul as an organ 93
86. Leaving behind karma in each sphere 95
87. Cellular penetration with the life forces 97
88. Polarities of the pelvis vs. head of male 98
89. Polarities of the pelvis vs. head of female 98
90. Gender differentiation in the pattern of arousal 100
91. Three phases of hormonal secretion 102
92. The female genital axis 103
93. Female pelvis as Grail with double vortex 105
94. Sound U as depiction 115
95. Eurythmy gesture of U 116
96. Life becomes a walk through a labyrinth 117
97. Preview and review 118
98. Temple with four pillars 120
99. Facial gestures 121
100. Carbon 122
101. Malpighi body 124
102. Imagination of living water 125
103. Bonding between physical and etheric 126
104. Enkido embracing the lion 128
105. Maya—illusion 129
106. Leaving karma behind 131

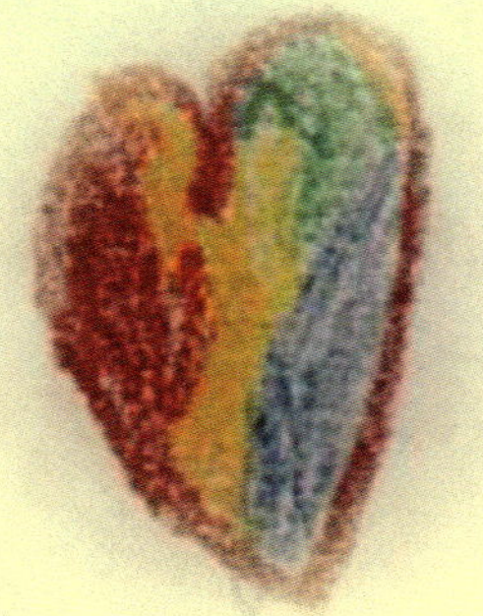